W9-AQF-107

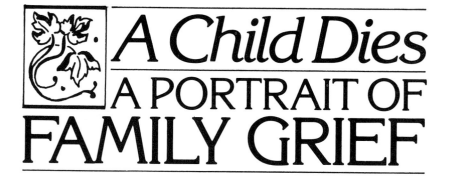

A Child Dies
A PORTRAIT OF
FAMILY GRIEF

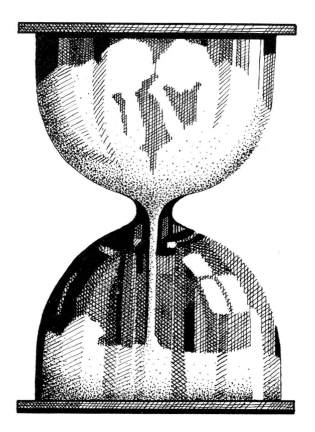

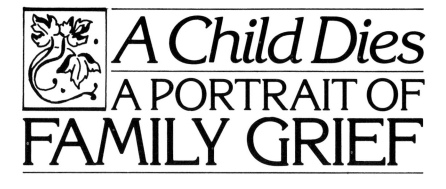

A Child Dies
A PORTRAIT OF
FAMILY GRIEF

Joan Hagan Arnold
Penelope Buschman Gemma
Foreword by
John E. Schowalter, MD

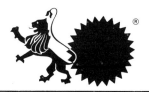

AN ASPEN PUBLICATION®
Aspen Systems Corporation
Rockville, Maryland
London
1983

Library of Congress Cataloging in Publication Data

Arnold, Joan Hagan.
A child dies.

Bibliography: p. 153
Includes index.
1. Children—Death—Psychological aspects.
2. Bereavement—Psychological aspects.
3. Parent and child.
4. Brothers and sisters.
5. Family psychotherapy.
I. Gemma, Penelope Buschman.   II. Title.
[DNLM: 1. Death—In infancy and childhood.
2. Attitude to death.   3. Grief.   4. Family.
                  BF 789.D4   A756c]
BF575.G7A76 1983   155.9'37   83-7132
                        ISBN: 0-89443-816-6

Publisher: John Marozsan
Editorial Director: Darlene Como
Executive Managing Editor: Margot G. Raphael
Printing and Manufacturing: Denise Hass
Cover Design: Lucinda C. Geist
Illustration: Lynn Harpell

Library of Congress Catalog Card Number: 83-7132
ISBN: 0-89443-816-6

Printed in the United States of America

2 3 4 5

To
Rick, Michael, and Matthew
J.H.A.

To
Pat, Jon, and Ben
P.B.G.

and To
The families who have shared their
memories with us

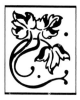 Contents

Foreword

YOU ARE EMBARKING ON A SPECIAL JOURNEY. THIS MAY SEEM like a curious statement to be made concerning a book about the death of children, but you will find that it is true.

Joan Hagan Arnold and Penny Buschman Gemma are unusual nurses and they have produced an unusual book. It provides a background of the meanings and manifestations of death and mourning; it discusses the ramifications of death at the various stages of childhood and adolescence; it describes the problems faced by the bereaved families and the opportunities, joys, and heartaches involved in working clinically in these special circumstances. This scope in itself is not unusual. What is striking, however, is the vibrancy of these women's understanding and caring, expressed in clear, touching, literate prose. These are not abstract theoreticians or followers of the latest psychosocial fad; they are caregivers who have spent their lives struggling with constant self-doubts and possible meanings of death during childhood.

The authors augment their extensive knowledge of the scientific literature on thanatology with the writings of others and statements of their own patients and their families. As a reader you feel you are in the hospital room, the clinic, and the home. Unlike some books on this subject, these transportations are not maudlin but appropriate aids to learning. The authors add yet another dimension to this subject through the use of thoroughly striking illustrations integrated harmoniously with the text that provide shocks of recognition leading to a reverie which mixes the reading with your own personal associations. These illustrations evoke time-enduring emotions.

Death is the one common link between all who have lived, are living, or will live. The authors make us realize that we are part of this chain and, as such, are able to help others who experience death before maturity. None of us is guaranteed long life, only a lifetime. This book helps us learn how to live life more fully through a more complete understanding of the meanings of death, which in turn allows us to be more understanding of our patients, our children, and ourselves.

John E. Schowalter, M.D.
Chief of Child Psychiatry
Yale Child Study Center
Yale University
New Haven, Connecticut

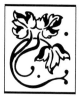 # *Preface*

Birth and death are monumental events, the cornerstones of existence. They are moments which evoke the greatest joy and sorrow. At these times onlookers, caregivers, and those experiencing the beginning or ending of a life come together in cohesion, understanding, support, and awe, or move apart in solitude, loneliness, and pain. Loss by death is inevitable in the experience of living. Through mourning we learn how to continue to live in the world with our losses. How we engage in this process seems to influence our potential for healthful living and relating with others.

The meaning of the death of a child to a family is the focus of this book. We contend that the experience of losing a child is special and like none other. Children are not supposed to die. The death of a child is a senseless injustice. A child's death—whether expected or unexpected, regardless of age and cause—is incomprehensible. Family members ache with their own powerlessness and vulnerability and live with emptiness. The family is never whole again because a significant member is missing.

When a child dies, silence often ensues and grows over the years. To speak about a child's death is considered unnatural, unwise, too threatening, too painful. How can families who ache and live with emptiness gain from silence? This book is an attempt to bring to the surface what has been silenced, in order to portray a child's death and the family's loss.

How can one become sensitive to the specialness of a child's death and continue to communicate compassion and understanding to the family? Is empathy possible in this instance? There are no answers to these questions. Rather, the authors seek to explore the issues that these questions raise and to draw child death into the realm of critical concerns and dilemmas that need to be faced openly. In our clinical practice, each has worked with families after a child's death and has been touched by the extent of their pain. We have been humbled by their strength to go on and learn to live without their child. Families have shared with us haltingly and openly when words and expressions could convey the fringes of their emotions and experiences. It is these expressions that we wish to make some ordering of, to speak for the families who have chosen to share their grief with us, so that the special meaning of a child's death can be told.

We had assumed that writing this book would be less difficult than it was. In the process we tapped into our own beings and experiences; we tried to sort out the similarities and differences in our impressions and approaches before we could attempt to analyze and present the family data in a clear and meaningful way. We then became recorders of this critical life event. The subject was painful to address. You may find the presentation of child death from a personal, experiential point of view, stripped of protective jargon, difficult to read.

We have focused on normal family bereavement following the death of a child member, that is, the wide range of grief reactions and behaviors that a family utilizes to express the experience of their loss. Purposefully we have refrained from presenting data dealing with individual and family psychopathology in response to the loss of a child but not because these reactions are not important and do not require attention. Indeed this topic deserves special consideration. Rather, we have sought to make visible the invisible, that is, the vast expanse of normal bereavement behavior after a child's death. While we have focused on child death spanning the period of infancy through adolescence, the family's process of grieving and living without occurs regardless of the age of the child member at death. Just as the family mourns the infant, the young child, and the adolescent, so does it mourn the adult child of any age. Grief for one's child knows no age limit.

It seemed that much of the clinical literature on parental bereavement did not adequately convey the intensity and depth of feelings experienced on the death of a child. There was little validation for what the families were experiencing. We turned to the artist for an accurate portrayal of this loss. Conveyed in a multitude of art forms was poignant validation for the timeless, boundless nature of the grief of parents. Tolstoy in *What Is Art?* wrote: "The business of art lies just in this, to make that understood and felt which, in the form of an argument, might be incomprehensible and inaccessible. Usually it seems to the recipient of a truly artistic impression that he knew the thing before but had been unable to express it" (1898).

For the many caregivers of bereaved families, this book was written in the hope that a deeper appreciation of the experience of child death will aid their coming together in support and understanding with families who have lost children. We wrote, too, for the many families who might benefit from sharing the experiences of others.

Reference

Tolstoy, L. [*What is art?*] (A. Maude, Trans.) Fair Lawn, N.J.: Oxford University Press, 1898.

Suggested Readings

Arnold, J.H. Child death and family bereavement: An exploration through the arts. *PRN: The Adelphi Report* (Project for Research in Nursing). Adelphi University, School of Nursing, 1980-1981, pp. 33-44.

Worby, D.Z. The death of the child in literature. *Mid-Hudson Language Studies,* 1978, *1,* 125-140.

Acknowledgments

IN THE PREPARATION OF A CLINICAL WORK OF THIS KIND, there is a chronology which can be recognized in the ordering of the acknowledgments. We began as clinicians deeply involved and committed to our patients and families.

My special thanks go to:

Donna O'Hare and *Jean Pakter*, New York City Department of Health for their invitation to join The Causes and Circumstances of Postneonatal Mortality project. My position permitted me to visit with families soon after the death of their infant child—an experience which altered the course of my life and fostered a commitment to representing them in some way.

Jean Pakter, Dominick DiMaio, Office of the Chief Medical Examiner, New York City and *Lucille Rosenbluth*, Medical and Health Research Association of New York City for the opportunity to serve as coordinator of the New York City Information and Counseling Program for Sudden Infant Death and for their guidance and support throughout. *Margaret O'Brien*, New York City Department of Health for her concern for the caregivers.

Geraldine Norris, United States Department of Health and Human Services for her gracious way and leadership.

Vera Michaels and *Christine Blenninger* for their lasting friendships and the joys of working together.

Arlene Casta for a decade of sharing, support, and for typing the final manuscript.

The Project for Research in Nursing, Adelphi University and to *Jacqueline Rose Hott* and *Pierre Woog*, Co-Coordinators for the opportunity to engage in a research project exploring creative literary sources in an effort to elucidate the nature of parents' grief. Special thanks to Pierre for the idea. This effort nurtured the subsequent unfolding of a search that led to the rich and diverse works of art included in our text.

June Rothberg, Dean and *M. Elaine Wittmann*, Undergraduate Program Director, Adelphi University and to all my colleagues at Adelphi for their ongoing support and for the delight they expressed in sharing in the process.

—*Joan H. Arnold*

My special thanks go to:

The many *families who have suffered the death of their children at Babies Hospital.* These families have shared and continue to share their grief and the ways in which they have begun to live without. These children and families have been my patients, my teachers, and my friends.

Jane McConville, a most wise and compassionate woman, the Associate Director of Nursing, Center for Women and Children, has given her warmth and encouragement and active support, making it possible for me to work, to learn, and to grow.

The *nursing staff of Babies Hospital*, a dynamic, changing group of women and men who care fiercely and competently, and lovingly for the children and their families.

William S. Langford, M.D., my wise mentor who shared his knowledge, skill, and vision.

Rodman Gilder, M.D., my trusted friend and teacher who gave ongoing clinical consultation, encouragement, and wisdom.

Robert Parkin, M.D., who sharing his family systems perspective, added another dimension to my clinical practice.

—*Penelope B. Gemma*

While formulating our ideas and thoughts into a presentation culminating in *A Child Dies: A Portrait of Family Grief* many individuals were helpful. We especially wish to acknowledge:

The *library staffs of both Adelphi University and Columbia University* for their help in the various literature searches and in the probing and looking for difficult to find references. Most special thanks to the Fine Arts Librarian, *Erica Doctorow* and to the Reference Librarian, *Carol Schroeder* at Adelphi.

The *children's librarian and reference staff at the Bryant Library* in Roslyn, New York.

Special fond thanks to *Sr. Mary Immaculate*, C.S.C., Professor of English at St. Mary's College, Notre Dame, Indiana, for her gift of *The Cry of Rachel,* a rich and powerful anthology of poetry about child death that we used liberally to illustrate our clinical impressions. Sr. Mary extended both her work and encouragement freely and graciously.

Anita Schorsch for sharing her wealth of knowledge of mourning art.

Mr. and Mrs. Frances Reisz for giving us their memories.

Phoebe Lloyd, Department of the History of Art, University of Pennsylvania, for sharing her dissertation full of the rich history of mourning art in this country.

Susan Williamson, for her friendship and perspective from many years of clinical practice.

Sherry Johnson-Soderberg, Assistant Professor, University of Illinois, for her interest and support.

John E. Schowalter, for his "Foreword" which captures in a few well chosen words what we struggled to say in many and for the validation he offers our work.

Lucinda Carbuto Geist, Lynn Harpell, and *Joan Harrison* for their artistry and keen sensitivity to this subject.

Darlene Como and *Margot G. Raphael* for their patience, expertise, and guidance in the preparation of our manuscript.

Peg Fumante, Millie Schifano and *Nancy Arnold* for their skill and thoughtfulness.

All our family members from whom we have grown and learned and to *our husbands and children* to whom this book is dedicated.

—*Joan H. Arnold and Penelope B. Gemma*

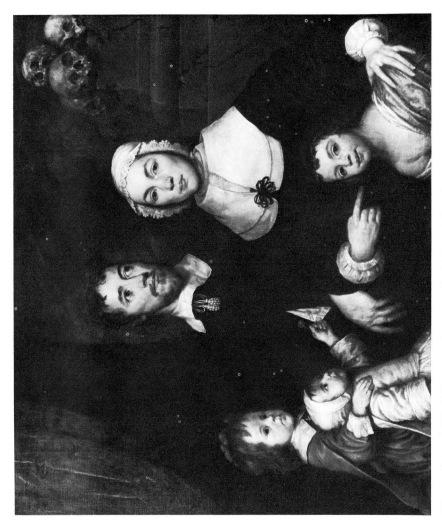

WILLIAM DOBSON (1611-1646). *Portrait Group, probably of the Streatfeild Family*. Oil on Canvas, 42 × 49½ in. (106.8 ×

The Streatfeild Family, William Dobson, British, 17th Century. A deceased child is not only included in this portrait of an English Puritan family, but is decidedly its subject. As the mother, tenderly affected, points to the child (draped unlike the other family members), the father casts his eyes on a death's head resting upon a cracked column. The family's hopes lie with the surviving children, the younger of whom, like infants in every age, tugs at his father's clothes for attention.

—Anita Schorsch*

*Reprinted from *Images of Childhood: An Illustrated Social History* by Anita Schorsch with permission from the author and The Main Street Press, 1979.

A Woman of the Mountain Keens Her Son[*]

Grief on the death, it has blackened my heart:
It has snatched my love and left me desolate,
Without friend or companion under the roof of my house
But this sorrow in the midst of me, and I keening.

As I walked the mountain in the evening
The birds spoke to me sorrowfully,
The sweet snipe spoke and the voiceful curlew
Relating to me that my darling was dead.

I called to you and your voice I heard not,
I called again and I got no answer,
I kissed your mouth, and O God how cold it was
Ah, cold is your bed in the lonely churchyard.

O green-sodded grave in which my child is,
Little narrow grave, since you are his bed,
My blessings on you, and thousands of blessings
On the green sods that are over my treasure

Grief on the death, it cannot be denied,
It lays low, green and withered together, —
and O gentle little son, what tortures me is
That your fair body should be making clay!

Padraic Pearse[*]
(1879-1916)

[*]Reprinted from *The 1916 Poets* with permission from Allen Figgis and Co. Ltd. Publishers, Dublin, Ireland.

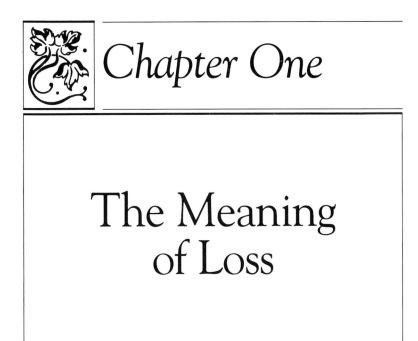

Chapter One

The Meaning
of Loss

Each substance of a grief hath twenty shadows.

—William Shakespeare
Richard II

LIFE IS FILLED WITH LOSS. LOSS IS INEVITABLE IN THE EXPERI-ence of living. It is inescapable. It is necessary for growth. In its broadest sense, the experience of loss is a universal, continuing process, part of the life process.

Often loss occurs without notice and may be as imperceptible or natural as in the changing of seasons, the shifting of tides, and the rotating of the earth. We lose yesterday and gain today. Loss is all around us, in all life forms, and within us—as cells are formed and die, as we leave childhood behind and move on to grow and change and die. Some losses carry with them deep emotional responses: sadness, hurt, bewilderment, rage, guilt, and fear. These emotions are felt regardless of how much is gained in growing and evolving. Loss leaves one feeling empty. Some empty spaces can never be filled, and some spaces that are filled still feel empty.

The process of life involves both gains and losses. A rhythmic pattern evolves; as time moves on and changes occur, one gets and gives up, one receives and gives away, one wins and one loses. We look forward to the gains; we delight in the joy of what is new and different—the freshness, specialness, uniqueness of each new experi-

3

ence or change within or about ourselves. Change, the process of growing and becoming, is preferred; it is valued highly. We celebrate our gains. But growing and becoming also mean moving away from, detaching, letting go, giving up, losing.

Losses are grieved. Dealing with feelings of loss does not come easily. Losses are not greeted readily; indeed, they may be feared and denied. We search and long for what we have lost. Loss hurts. It is the hurt in life that we hope to soothe, hope to quiet and cover, hope to repair and recover from as quickly as possible. It is difficult to welcome and accept losses; rather, we seek more to hold on to what we have.

Loss has other meanings apart from the natural flow of life's energy and pattern. Loss also means being stripped, robbed, divested, denuded. To suffer loss means to undergo deprivation; to be depleted and bereaved; to be apart from, wanting, lacking, and cut off; to be dissipated, consumed, gone forever. Loss is to have no longer. Loss evokes feelings of horror in the human experience.

Loss is experienced through death. Death can occur instantaneously, in that instant forever changing our lives. Yet nothing else remains still. The rest of life continues. In truth, one who is living is also dying all the time. We have come to recognize and treat life and death as if they are opposite, incompatible states of existence or opposing ends of the continuum that we call the life cycle, a start versus a finish. They are not at war with one another but are part of each other. Living and dying, growing and losing are one process. We grieve continually. The nature and extent of our grief vary in intensity and meaning; sometimes we are more conscious of grief and can cope with it better than at other times.

We cannot achieve a state of resolution because loss through death is permanent and our grief continuous. The pain of loss is difficult to deal with for that loss will never be recovered. There is no way to return once one has moved on. There is no way to recapture, to relive. There is no way to grow in relationships once they are gone. What do we do about our losses? What do we do with our feelings? We bury them, live with their memory, try to forget, try to hold on in some way to what was, and idealize. There are specified times when it is all right to expose our true feelings, but generally they must remain private, stored in the depths of our experience. We move away from persons who share their losses too willingly or openly.

Losing a loved one and grieving for him transcend familial, societal, and cultural boundaries. Although the significance of the experience may be generalizable, the management of the experience may be quite different from one family and cultural group to another (Spradley & Phillips, 1972, p. 519). How we recognize the loss, how we measure the importance of loss, how we respond, what we deem permissible in expression, and how we ritualize expressions and behaviors are among the differences that set us apart.

Loss produces change in the life of the individual, family, and society. The impact of loss depends on its nature and scope. Often the pain of loss comes with the need to give up that someone or something precious or that part of ourselves that has been taken away. When someone is taken from us, we do not let go willingly. There is a peculiar physical violence to loss by death, a sudden and powerful force. We do not participate in the letting go; rather, we feel as if the person for whom we long has been stripped, ripped, torn, and severed from us and we are left to feel separate and unconnected, cut off. "What is Life? It departs covertly. Like a thief Death took him" (Gunther, 1949, p. 111). One remains in pain and sadness with the problems of reordering one's existence, often with little recognition and support.

Though our losses may signify profound and painful times for us, others may be unaware of how deeply hurt we are. We may feel out of synchrony with the movement around us, but the motion does not stop for us—nothing stands still when death occurs.

We have come to legitimize this process of dealing with sorrow by calling it *grieving, mourning,* or *bereavement.* Much attention has been devoted to this working through of loss. Attempts are made to record and analyze the behaviors of the bereaved. Commonalities in experience are searched for to develop a schema to help others study and understand the progression of this state and to delineate boundaries for normal and abnormal behavior. But grief cannot be contained. It knows no boundaries. It defies classification and categorization. Grief is too large, too complex; grief is everywhere and cannot be reduced or ordered. To talk about grief means accepting first that words can

FALL 1968

He's dead; and the pain is immense.
Your heart goes numb in the knowledge
that he is no more.

You daren't ask why he, of all people,
had to die—for you know
there is no answer.

And in your shock,
You notice the world doesn't stop
turning
even though he is gone.

> Glen Mitchell Gittelson
> (April 27, 1956—May 25, 1971)
> *A Sugared Bitter Tart*

Glen wrote this poem at the age of 12,
three years before his death.

neither describe adequately its emotions nor convey its pervasive pain. Putting grief into words reduces its power; it is an empty effort to contain it. Grief is limitless and powerful. But we must talk to each other about our grief and acknowledge that we can never know for sure another's pain. Each person's response to loss is an expression of one's own way of coping; no one way is better than another. Each person makes meaning out of loss. We share what we can. Sharing helps to bind us by deepening our relationships, reducing the isolation that we feel.

Mourning is a process that involves coming to terms with the loss, learning to live without, learning to live with emptiness, to make meaning out of deprivation, to rejoin and carry on differently. We long for what we have lost. We search for meaning and significance from the pain and emptiness that we feel. We need to order events and circumstances so that they become comprehensible, explicable, rational, and reasonable. We wish for what could have been. We wonder why, and we feel deprived and angry, empty and powerless. Regardless of our hopes and desires, of the promises and commitments that we make, life will not be returned. What is gone through death cannot be regained, reclaimed, reconnected. We must learn to cope without, to adjust to the changes, to accept the emptiness, to integrate, to move on, without.

It is difficult to live with feeling lonely, separate, and unconnected. When one is bereaved, one feels out of touch with the mainstream, different, unable to connect. One feels stigmatized, deprived, and angry for being selected to suffer. One wonders why. Rarely is there rhyme or reason. It is unfair, unjust that life deals out such pain for us to bear. There is little recognition of the bereaved. It is expected that one should mourn, but mourn "appropriately," that is, within the specifications of acceptable behavior: to cry, but only so much; to sulk and stare blankly, but only for so long; to feel helpless and unable to participate, but only for a short time. We are expected to get up, pull ourselves together, tuck our pain and agony away, stop the flow of tears. We are to live again, to behave as though grief is over and behind us. Traffic moves, appointments are kept, and, as time passes, fewer people ask about feelings because one is expected to participate again. Yet for the mourners it is as though life has stopped within. As

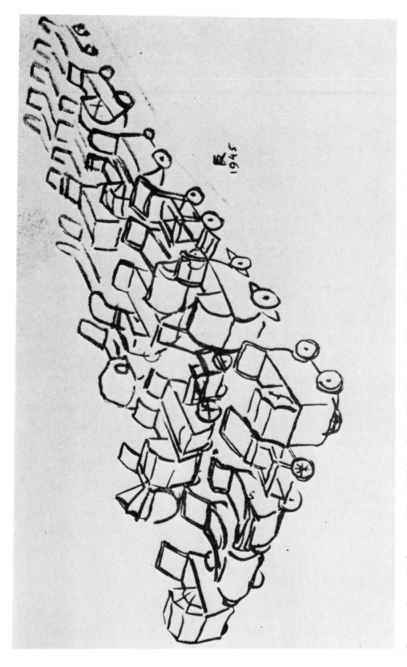

FRANCIS REISZ. *Kinderwagen.* Hôpital Bichat, Paris, 1945. Tusche auf Papier, 13 × 20.8 cm (Reprinted with permission from the artist. From *Temoignages sur Auschwitz*, edition de L'Amicale Des Déportés D'Auschwitz, dessins de Francois Reisz, Paris, 1945)

8

"Kinderwagen" commemorates the death of untold numbers of children of Gypsy families imprisoned in Auschwitz and exterminated with their families in 1944. Francis Reisz recalls the loss he and other survivors felt when early one morning the Gypsy campsite was silent as the smoke from the gas chambers filled the air. Rows of baby carriages, once full of joy and life now empty, were efficiently lined up at an exit from the gas chamber building. (The artist and his wife now reside in New York City.)

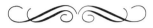

mourners we feel that we too have died; death moves in to occupy and possess us, to join with us and be part of us.

The experience of loss erupts feelings associated with previous losses and previous pain. We reach into the past to childhood and feel hurts of long ago. What is lost throughout life is longed for, searched for. We wish to reclaim and to make ourselves whole again, filled with the tenderness and affection of relationships that are gone. It is difficult to let go. Yet letting go allows us to grow and change without attachments that might hold us still and leave us feeling anger, frustration, and guilt.

We attempt to make meaning out of loss. We attribute special reasons or attempt to answer the whys in ways that foster our ability to cope and acknowledge our losses. We need to order things, analyze, organize, and perhaps tuck losses into the back of our minds, as far away as possible. Individual, family, and societal defenses and religious beliefs and patterns combine to facilitate living without. We cope in the best way that we can. We long for and linger in helplessness and sadness until some inner energy mobilizes to carry us beyond the experience of loss.

Loss connects one human being with another. Loss is a human phenomenon. Experiencing loss and finding meaning in it bind caretaker to sufferer. Loss is an equalizer.

The loss of a child is a loss like none other. Child death is the death of innocence, the death of the most vulnerable, the delicate, the dependent, the needy. The death of a child signifies the loss of the future, of hopes and dreams, of new strength, and of perfection.

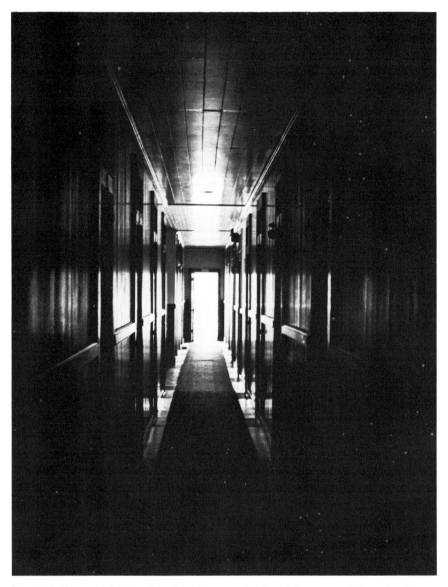

Empty Hall. Photograph by Karen Dusenbery. (Courtesy of St. Louis Information and Counseling Program for Sudden Infant Death, from a brochure developed by consortium representatives of six SIDS Information and Counseling Projects, supported by the Bureau of Health and Human Services, Office of Maternal and Child Health. Unpublished.)

For parents, the agony of losing a child is unparalleled. When their child dies, the parents die; a vital part of them has been severed. Parents grieve the lost child for the rest of their lives, never to be whole again. A parent's grief is forever. Only memories remain.

Loss leaves memories. Memories cannot be taken from us. Memories soothe and comfort us. They are ours alone in solitude and ours to share with others if we choose. Memories bring us recognition of what we had. They stand as an unshakable account of our past. These imprints bring joy, sorrow, and pain. We can shape and form our memories to give us comfort, approval, and support, or remorse and guilt. Memories alter in time, perhaps becoming idealized, perhaps vague. But memories belong to us. We keep close to us, with us, memories of those whom we love and have lost.

> *. . . death eventually separates everyone*
> *from each other. It is only the vividness*
> *of memory that keeps the dead alive forever.*
>
> —John Irving
> *The World According to Garp*

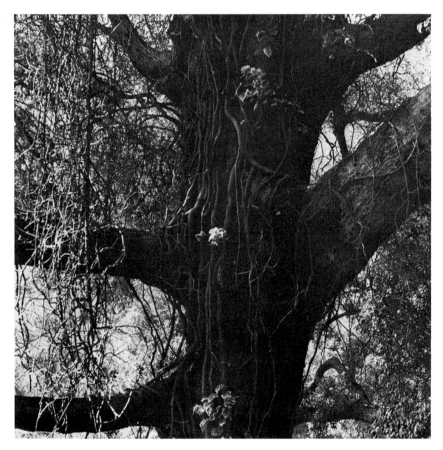

Mossy Tree. Photograph by Karen Dusenbery. (Courtesy of St. Louis Information and Counseling Program for Sudden Infant Death.)

References

Gunther, J. *Death be not proud: A memoir.* New York: Harper & Row, 1949.

Irving, J. *The world according to Garp.* New York: E.P. Dutton, 1978.

Spradley, J.P., and Phillips, M. Culture and stress: A quantitative analysis. *American Anthropologist,* 1972, *4*, 518-529.

Suggested Readings

Aries, P. *Western attitudes toward death: From the Middle Ages to the present.* Baltimore: The Johns Hopkins University Press, 1974.

Kearns, M. *Kathe Kollwitz: Woman and artist.* New York: The Feminist Press, 1976.

Lewis, C.S. *A grief observed.* New York: Bantam Books, Inc., 1976.

Lindemann, E. *Beyond grief: Studies in crisis intervention.* New York: Jason Aronson, 1979.

Moustakas, C.E. *Loneliness.* Englewood Cliffs, N.J.: Prentice-Hall, Inc., 1961.

Schoenberg, B., Gerber, I., Wiener, A., Kutscher, A.H., Peretz, D., and Carr, A.C. (Eds.). *Bereavement: Its psychosocial aspects.* New York: Columbia University Press, 1975.

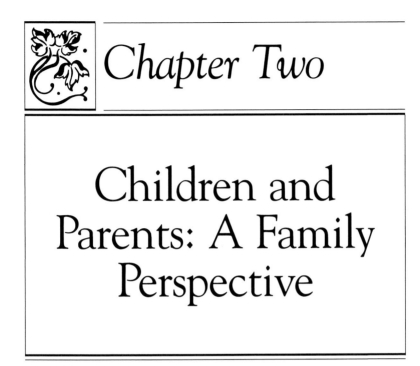

Chapter Two

Children and Parents: A Family Perspective

T O APPRECIATE THE IMPACT OF CHILD DEATH ON THAT CLUS-
ter of persons living together, the complex system that we term the
family, we must stand back and look carefully at the whole as well as at
some components and qualities. Each family system is unique and
possesses characteristics that are different from all others. Families
differ in their culture, history, and tradition as well as in patterns of
communication, work, and organization. The culture, history, and
traditions of a family are its links to the persons and experiences that
are part of a past flow of life and provide for that family the special
flavor that comes from the blending and meshing of ethnic back-
grounds, patterns of speech, values, mores, the true and distorted
stories of how the family grew, who was born and died, and the ways
in which the family celebrates its special events and times. The
culture, history, and tradition are connecting points for a family and
provide a means for constancy and continuity in the face of social
change and upheaval.

Composition differs from family group to family group. One may
be the traditional nuclear family including mother, father, and children, or the group may include the parents, children, and some

members of the extended family. Social changes are reflected in the increased number of single-parent families with one parent assuming primary responsibility for the nurture and care of the children. If parents are separated or divorced, the second parent may share in some way the financial and emotional responsibility for child care. This may be assumed regularly and consistently or erratically. An adult companion of the single parent may be invested in the care of the children. This companion may be a relatively stable presence over a long period or may be replaced. Extended family members, friends, and child care workers may also assume some responsibility for the children.

Assumed and assigned roles differ from family to family. Parents traditionally provide care and share the responsibilities. In many families there no longer is rigid adherence to traditional male-female duties and assigned tasks. More often the roles shift according to need. Many mothers have reentered or have never left a field of employment. Fathers may provide care for the child or, if they are fully employed, may share in child care and in the other tasks of maintaining a home.

There is tremendous strength in the fabric of some families, in which bonds and loyalties are firm, conveying warmth and a sense of support to members in need. There are others whose fabric is weak and torn, whose members extend their network outside the family to look for and find sources of strength.

The degree to which members of a family are connected to one another but separate from each other is an important measure of function. There are families where the connectedness supports growth and fosters the process of individuation necessary for the child member to separate and assume some responsibility for his own person, for the decisions that he must make, and for how he will live with the family history. There are others who enmesh and entangle members, impeding or preventing the child's growth and ability to move on.

ON BEING A PARENT

Within the family system are the special relationships between and among family members. A primary one is that between parent and child. It is comparable to no other relationship between human beings in its uniqueness and complexity. There is a connectedness between parent and child that has its roots in the biological and emotional connections and attachments that precede birth; it grows as the parent begins to know and care for the child. One's child is a part of the self and a separate self all at once. A child is a parent's link to the future, the guarantee that life will go on. The parent's life is embodied in this child.

The relationship of parent to child is characterized by its potential for intimacy. The child who is conceived by the parents or adopted into their family is watched and listened to until his breath sounds are familiar, his sleeping-waking patterns known, and his needs and the ways in which he makes them known are understood.* As the child grows, the parent can be an active participant in the developmental process, encouraging and fostering the innate ability to learn, to acquire and master new skills, and to grow. With the growing is the recognition of separateness, the realization that the child, who was physiologically part of the parent, remains emotionally part of the parent but becomes in some respects a stranger as he grows and unfolds.

Characterizing the parent-child relationship is the responsibility of parent to child and conversely in more subtle ways from child to parent as the child grows. The parent creates the child's life and is primarily responsible for sustaining and protecting it, shielding it from the dangers, actual and imagined, that threaten it. There is vulnerability in the relationship, the potential for grave hurt and disappointment. The parent is threatened by what might happen to the child if he is not vigilant in his protection. The child might be hurt, maimed, or killed—taken unexpectedly.

---

*Note: This book follows the standard practice of using a masculine pronoun wherever the pronoun refers to either or both sexes. Feminine pronouns appear only where antecedents are exclusively female.

A power and a powerlessness exist in the relationship between parent and child. There is power to determine certain decisions and directions when the child is young and a powerlessness to prevent all harm, protect from all threats.

Ambivalence characterizes the relationship as both positive and negative feelings emerge in response to the child. The parent lives with guilt when feeling anger toward and disapproval of the child.

To become a parent, to grow into parenthood is a most difficult task. Becoming a parent is a process that occurs over a lifetime. It begins with one's own experience of being parented, the quality of the parents or parent surrogates who rendered care. Parents draw on their own experience as they had been nurtured, loved, and cared for. They may agree to make changes in child-rearing practices (the techniques and strategies used to promote behavioral changes), but the foundation laid firmly and squarely in childhood is remembered and drawn on. One must be nurtured in order to nurture.

There is a time to begin to prepare for parenting—consciously during pregnancy or while awaiting the arrival of an adopted child— a time to imagine oneself a parent, to practice, to gain skills and information, to make room physically and emotionally for the small person who will become such a central focus in one's life. There are many ways to prepare for the arrival of a child from the reordering of one's work and social schedules, travel and leisure plans, to the shifting of furniture and space, to the purchasing of items necessary for care, to the calling on friends and family whose experience, wisdom, and comfort with children are sought after. Being a parent or parenting, doing the responsible work of a parent, means establishing initially an environment in which a child can grow, building a relationship that fosters growth while providing for the safety and protection of the child.

Parental advocacy of the child supports him and allows him to move away from parent and home, feeling worthwhile and loved and strong enough to stand apart. Parenting means letting go, giving up, accepting the reality that as the child grows and changes, he can never return to where he was. Parenting is losing and accepting the losses inherent in growth.

You may give them your love but not your thoughts,
For they have their own thoughts.
You may house their bodies but not their souls,
For their souls dwell in the house of tomorrow, which
you cannot visit, not even in your dreams. . . .

Kahlil Gibran
"On Children," *The Prophet**

*Reprinted from *The Prophet,* by Kahlil Gibran, by permission of Alfred A. Knopf, Inc. Copyright 1923 by Kahlil Gibran and renewed 1951 by Administrators C. T. A. of Kahlil Gibran Estate . . . and Mary G. Gibran.

While becoming a parent and parenting, the parent develops certain expectations for the child—some realistic, some based on his own experiences—wishes, hopes and dreams. The parent shares and gives of his own experience and actively plans for and with his child.

ON BEING A CHILD

In each of us is a child. This child is the composite of experience and memory that we carry with us. It is that portion of us influenced by temperament, shaped by the relationships with our families and the patterns used by our parents in their parenting of us, the special needs that were met and unmet, the important developmental issues and life experiences that we negotiated and continue to negotiate that link us to others. The child part is always with us, interpreting and responding to the world and to those with whom we live.

We identify the child in the adult—in ourselves and in others. Conversely we see ourselves in our children and we are more or less comfortable with the part of ourselves that we see or wish to see in our children, as if the same eyes, nose, mouth, or temperamental bent may symbolize the intimacy, the closeness, the connectedness between parent and child, a continuation of our own existence through the child. It is the unknown in the child, the qualities that unfold as the child develops that surprise and excite. The parent recognizes the child as a little stranger as well as someone whom no one else knows better or can comfort or delight.

The child grows and changes in response to the amount and level of nurturing and protection that is experienced in the family and community. The growth process is constantly in motion. The developmental potential in each child is essentially unknown. Measurements are crude at best. There is no way of predicting how far genetic, temperamental, and constitutional limits can be stretched if the environmental factors that mold and influence are supportive of growth. The child grows within the family.

This developmental potential exists in every part of the child's being, in cognition, in emotion, in creative spirit, in socialization as well as in the physical body. As he grows and as the growth is supported, the child acquires new skills. He shifts from a concrete, limited appreciation of his world to an expanded view that allows him to think conceptually and reason more fully. The child is curious and asks questions to acquire knowledge. Even before this cognitive shift occurs, the well-nurtured child can move from an egocentric world view to one that includes and is affected by the thoughts and feelings of parents, siblings, and important friends.

The creative potential in every child is less well known. That imaginative spark can be kindled until it bursts into the flame of an idea, a symphony, a beautiful work of art, a wonderfully funny joke. In some children the potential can be recognized early. In others it becomes evident as the child grows. It unfolds and there are no bounds.

Children embody the hopes and dreams of their parents. They are the parents' link to their past childhoods and their future existence. They are unique persons, separate from their families but connected in firm and lasting ways.

SOCIETY'S VIEW OF THE CHILD

There is an apparent contradiction in our society about the value of the child. Although recognized as valuable and in need of nurture, protection, and stimulation in order to grow, legislative and societal sanctions can hinder and prevent this growth. Our society, which claims to value the child, through its practices often neglects to protect its children. While the child clearly has value to his family, parents, and siblings, his place in society at large is limited and in question. Our society seems ambivalent toward its children, with lip service given to the importance of today's children being tomorrow's responsible adults while simultaneously focus shifts away from programs and funding geared to improving the lot of children and families.

This discrepancy is important to appreciate. The child should be protected, nurtured, and properly socialized by the family because of his future value as a contributor to society. As a child, his contribution to society is considered minimal, his place quite unimportant,

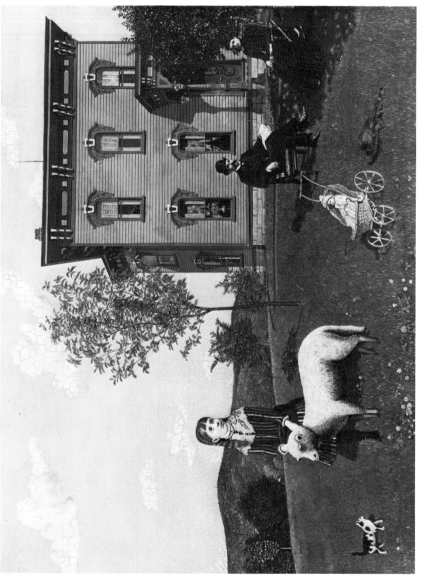

EDWIN ROMANZO ELMER, American, 1850-1923. *Mourning Picture*, 1890, Oil on Canvas, 28 × 36 in. (71.1 × 91.5 cm.) (Courtesy of

. . . Edwin Romanzo Elmer's painting of 1889 achieves a complete fusion of the living with the dead. The Elmers had one adored child, Effie. They lived in a house Edwin had built before their marriage. After Effie's sudden death, her mother's grief was so extreme she could no longer bear to see children and would not remain in the empty house. Before they moved away, however, Edwin Elmer took up brush and canvas to commemorate their life together. He painted Effie, her pets and toys, his wife and himself in mourning dress, all in front of their house. Elmer's work, an end product of the posthumous mourning portrait genre, most dramatically illustrates the American wish to mitigate death's finality through art.

—Phoebe Lloyd*

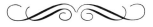

perhaps because the child is valued little. Thus the family is responsible for the child whom it values. His life is to be preserved and sustained until he can take an active, equal part in adult society. When he dies, the family has in some way failed in its task. When a child dies, society hardly provides for and supports the family in mourning.

There was a time when child death, although devastating, was expected. Death was commonplace and a child's death not unnatural but one of the many burdens that a family was forced to accept. Disease was rampant and children were particularly vulnerable. Families were larger, perhaps to protect from the harshness of life so that parents could be assured that some children would remain. Children died as frequently as adults did; life expectancy was a fraction of what we know today.

Those who mourned were recognized by their symbols and actions. Today the mourner is anonymous. Funerals are recognized for the ritualistic and therapeutic value. Families and friends gather but disperse soon after. There is little time to mourn, and little recognition is given the bereaved. Shortly after a death, one is expected to

*Reprinted from Phoebe Lloyd, "Posthumous Mourning Portraiture," in Martha V. Pike and Janice Gray Armstrong, *A Time to Mourn: Expressions of Grief in Nineteenth Century America* (Stony Brook, N.Y.: The Museums at Stony Brook, 1980), p. 85.

gather together the pieces of life that remain and resume the routines almost as though no lapse had occurred. There is social pressure against the prolonged and public expression of personal grief. One is expected to wipe away any sign of acute mourning, to reduce and cover intense emotion, and to regain control—as though to deny the very existence of one's loss.

When a child dies, this urgency to wipe away is more exaggerated. The social pressure toward denial of loss becomes pressure to deny one's pain, sorrow, and loneliness and therefore finally to deny the very existence of this precious and loved child. What is it about a child's death that makes parents part of an underground of mourners? For the most part, the mourners who grieve for their children are alone, often isolated. The armband and mourning garb no longer exist. Who is to know which of us has lost a child? The bereaved, silently longing for their children, are all about us.

The horror of a child's death has become so frightening to us that we seek to protect ourselves—as though the germs of death could be disseminated as easily as they were in centuries past. We fear con-tamination, if only in an emotional sense; we do not want to be touched by the demon who takes children to their death. This is a time when children are not expected to die. We choose to battle with death, expecting to conquer it with our abilities and strengths. We marvel at medical knowledge and technology and expect miracles. We believe in our knowledge and machines so much that when death wins, we find it painful to accept defeat. Defeat seems impossible, unbelievable. We exclaim, "No, it cannot be!" and refuse to accept its finality. The time in which we live presents these many dilemmas for the mourner.

A child's life is precious and each child's death a significant, agonizing blow. Parents grieve forever and live with the memories that they have of their child—each memory vivid and dear, painful and comforting.

The death of a child member affects individual members and the whole family system. There may be a resultant alteration in family structure and in the members' roles. The strengths and values of the family may be questioned as members turn to or away from the family for support and comfort.

Death of a child member becomes an important identifying piece of information about the family. It is woven into its history and into the everyday operation of members' lives. The child who has died continues to be a family member after death. Parents are forever parents of a dead child as well as of the surviving children. The dead child lives in memory. The family grieves for him and remembers him with little comfort and support from the society around them. The family of a child who dies lives without that child's physical presence and actual contributions but with memories, wishes, dreams, and hopes.

Suggested Readings

Aries, P. *Centuries of childhood.* New York: Alfred A. Knopf, 1962.

Lloyd, P. *Death and American painting: Charles Willson Peale to Albert Pinkham Ryder.* Unpublished doctoral dissertation. The City University of New York, 1980.

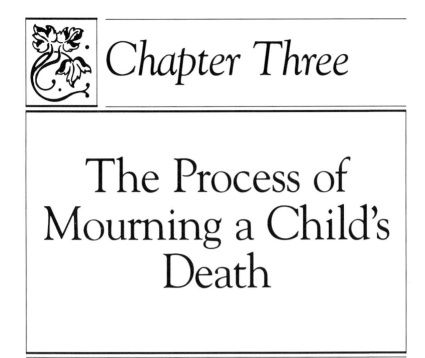

Chapter Three

The Process of Mourning a Child's Death

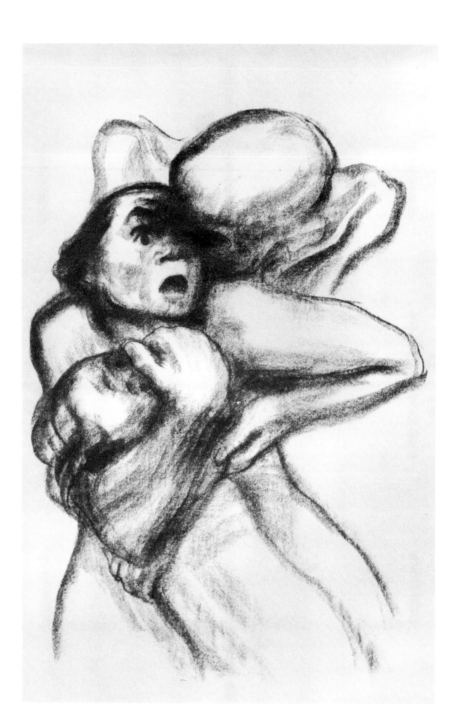

KATHE KOLLWITZ, *Death Reaches for a Child*. Lithograph, 1934. (Photograph courtesy Galerie St. Etienne, New York)

Ah woe is me! Winter is come and gone. But grief returns with the revolving year.

—Percy Bysshe Shelley
Adonais

T HERE IS NO RELATIONSHIP LIKE THAT OF PARENT AND CHILD. It is unique and special. It is incomparable in its complexities, responsibilities, and vulnerabilities. The bond between parent and child is so powerful that its strength endures time, distance, and strife. Despite this strength, this relationship between parent and child can be threatened. A child's life can end.

Parents live with vulnerability and dread, knowing that their child can be taken from them, that their child can die. This is an everpresent, silent fear of parents. The threat of the possible death of one's child enters dreams and fantasies. Parents continuously battle this sense of dread and try to quiet and hide it in the deepest well of their being. As it creeps into consciousness, it paralyzes and leaves one impotent to prevent, alter, or forbid it. The threat is that death can occur regardless of the degree of parental caring and carefulness. Parents cannot anticipate all events, reverse or change the course of time and circumstance capable of inflicting hurt and even death.

To be a parent is to be vulnerable. A parent's ability to protect is limited. This absence of control is horrifying. Parents ache with the knowledge that their greatest vulnerability lies in their inability to shield their child completely from death. Death is always possible, lurking, unforeseeable, final, and irreversible.

To be a parent is to be responsible. Central to all parenting responsibilities is the sustenance and maintenance of the child's life. Surrounding this core responsibility are loving and sharing, giving and guiding, believing and supporting. But the very essence of parenting is assuring life, protecting, keeping safe. A child can die in an instant—suddenly, by accident, violence, or illness—or after long and painful days of suffering. Death may be unforeseen or known and anticipated. Regardless of the time that it takes or the form that it chooses, parents are helpless; death repudiates their wish to protect and rejects their plea of "not me, please not me!"

No loss is as significant as the loss of a child to a parent. Children are from us and always remain part of us; they are connected to us. As their lives unfold, there is the potential for the realization of the parents' hopes and dreams. The child is the future. Parents are left unwhole without the child. The dead child's space remains empty. The parents' emptiness is part of their very being.

A parent's grief is grief for the separate person that has filled life with uncountable experiences and brought comfort, peace and love, and grief for the empty space within, the space that cannot be occupied by anyone or anything again. The child who occupied that space, a vital part of the self, has been cut out, torn, or ripped away; the loss is physically violent and painful as the child's life is severed from the parent. The body compensates to cope with this loss. Grieving, the healing process, attempts to seal and protect the space of the child for the sake of the parent's integrity and to preserve the relationship with the child.

FEELING LESS THAN WHOLE

On the death of a child, the parent feels less than whole. The sense of self is diminished. The parent's self-esteem is shattered, for the foundation of this significant role has been shaken. The longing for the child and the feeling of emptiness may last a lifetime. A parent grieves forever when a child dies. Although the magnitude

ON THE DEATH OF HIS BABY SON

I will never be able to stop my tears.
And the day is far off when I will
Forget this cruel day.
Why could we not have died with him?
His little clothes still hang on his rack
His milk is still by his bed.
Overcome, it is as though life had left us.
We lie prostrate and insensible all day.
I am no longer young enough
To try to understand what has happened.
I was warned of it in a dream.
No medicine would have helped.
Even if it had been heaped mountain high.
The disease took its course inexorably.
It would be better for me if I took
A sword and cut open my bowels.
They are already cut to pieces with sorrow.
I realize what I am doing
And try to come to myself again,
But I am exhausted and helpless,
Carried away by excess of sorrow.

Su Tung P'o (1036-1101)
Translated from the Chinese
by Kenneth Rexroth *

and intensity of grief will change with time and events, it does continue. It may provide comfort and solace; it may reduce one to despair, to tears of loneliness and longing, or to feelings of hopelessness and worthlessness; it may bring joy in remembering the child and the love shared. A child's death is unnatural and unjust. When a child dies, this loss is not resolved; rather, the parent continues to grieve, and grieving becomes a way of learning to live without the dead child and with the memories of that child. Death ends the child's life but it does not sever the bond between parent and child. They remain connected regardless of death, and grieving becomes a way of keeping connected. Searching and yearning for the child to reunite and reestablish a living connection continue despite the fact of death. Grieving is keeping memories alive and continuing to relate and maintain a place in the family for the dead child.

The nature of grief on the death of a child cannot be adequately described; no schema can contain it. Its breadth and depth defy description. Grieving is a continuous process, with peaks, valleys, and plateaus. It is a complex process that is bound to the individual who grieves uniquely like none other. Many have carefully attempted to define the process of bereavement, identifying major tasks, steps, and stages. We know little of the time grief takes. How can we describe something so profound that clouds our minds and numbs our senses? In retrospect we try to make sense of it; by listening to others, we try to capture the essence of their painful messages.

Parental grief is boundless, complex, and everchanging. It cannot be categorized or ordered, nor can it be justly described. It is lifelong and compounded by previous losses and how they were dealt with. With time the pain of grief will lessen; one could not survive if the pain continued to be as intense as it was at the death. However, without warning and often synchronized with special events or remembrances of the child, the pain returns as if the death had just occurred. The valley is deep and wide, the emptiness is pervasive. Grieving the death of one's child becomes a process of learning to live without the child and embarking on a journey to search for meaning where there is none and answers to unanswerable questions: Why did my child die? Why me? What made this happen to me?

The questioning is endless. Self-blame, guilt, and feelings of failure can plague parents, who know that they must have been responsible in some way for the death. Self-accusations undermine all logical explanations. No reason is sufficient to explain the death of a child. There is no justice or justification in a child's death.

Memories help to soothe the pain. They offer comfort as the dead child is remembered and as the attachment to the parent is maintained. Parental grief is not easily explained, not even by the many theorists proposing models for describing and explaining bereavement. In fact, normal parental grief may approximate accepted descriptions of pathological mourning. Normal, healthy grief responses for parents faced with their child's death may appear extreme, too intense, even bizarre and too long. The parent as well as the concerned observer feel the lack of guideposts to clarify natural versus disturbed responses, the range in expression of parental grief is so vast.

Parents may describe their profound emptiness or feeling of deadness inside. There is a senselessness to life; it could end and it would not matter, for the reason for living is gone. The injustice of losing one's child leads some parents to challenge beliefs and values while others hold to their beliefs as a stabilizing force. Expectations of what is reasonable, good, and just in life are changed.

The death of their child assaults the parents' sense of self-esteem and leaves them to question their ability to care for their surviving or subsequent children. There is no middle road; the perception is that any event or problem will inevitably result in death. The parent feels less a person, less a parent, less integrated, less able to function, less able to make decisions and judgments, a diminished self. For some, the child may have been the only source of pleasure and gratification in a life of deprivation and wanting. The child was the embodiment of the parents' wishes, hopes, and dreams.

Parents give their children what they most wanted for themselves and never had. When the child dies, there is no recipient for those special gifts. Parents continue to give their love, wishing for a response and finding none. The relationship is no longer reciprocal. Death only takes away. It forbids the continuation of sharing in each other's lives. It denies growth in the relationship. The future is only

PIETA *

Once only, with one hand,
Your mother in farewell
Touched you. I cannot tell,
I cannot understand

A thing so dark and deep,
So physical a loss:
One touch, and that was all
She had of you to keep.

* 8 lines of 'Pieta' reprinted with the permission from Angus and Robertson (UK) Ltd. from James McAuley's *Collected Poems*.

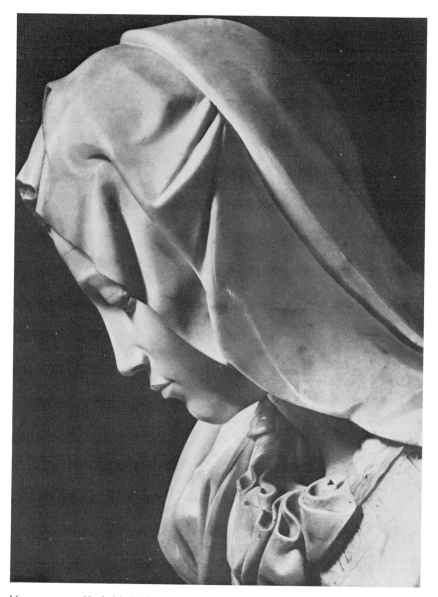

MICHELANGELO. *Head of the Madonna.* (Owner: Vatican. By courtesy of Rev. Fabbrica Di S. Pietro and Phaidon Press Limited, Oxford, England)

what could have been, the dreams of what might have been. The memories are of yesterday so that the parent is denied the joy of continuing to grow and share in the life of this child.

ANGER AND LONELINESS

The parent is left with anger. Anger may be felt toward the dead child for leaving, and this may be difficult or impossible to acknowledge—it becomes woven into peripheral or unrelated situations. The parent may feel anger toward the spouse, in some way blaming the partner for the child's death. Others involved in the child's world—physicians, teachers, babysitters—may be blamed. Anger is also directed outwardly toward families with children for their happiness and toward families who do not realize the treasure that they hold. Anger is also directed within in the form of self-blame, self-hatred, and shame. This inner rage may manifest itself as depression, violence, and self-destruction.

Grief is solitary. Even when surrounded by other people, the parent is alone. The normal patterns in relationship are disrupted. A strange dysynchrony pervades all of living. It is as though life moves on and the parent is left dazed and out of step, out of harmony with the pace of life and relationships. The parent is alone in grief and out of touch so that the magnitude of the loss cannot be communicated or acknowledged. There are no words to express the parent's feelings. Language is inadequate. The cries of grief cannot be heard. For some the cries of grief cannot be put into words. They may try to contain their feelings deep inside fearing the enormity of their grief, as though the volcano within may erupt.

The parent searches for some remnant of the child. Families may choose to leave the child's room as it was when he died, as though to preserve it, so that his memory and place will be lasting, to maintain his presence should this not be real and he return. Parents may forbid any dismantling or putting away of the child's things for a time. The room may be a place in which to cry or to feel the presence of the child by being in his space. The room may be sealed off like a museum or shrine, not entered because it is too agonizing to accept the loss.

The Recall*

The night was dark when she went away,
   and they slept.
The night is dark now, and I call for her
"Come back, my darling; the world is asleep;
   and no one would know, if you came for
   a moment while stars are gazing at stars."

She went away when the trees were in bud
   and the spring was young,
Now the flowers are in high bloom and I call,
"Come back, my darling. The children gather
   and scatter flowers in reckless sport.
   And if you come and take one little blossom
   no one will miss it."

Those that used to play are playing still,
   so spendthrift is life
I listen to their chatter and call,
"Come back, my darling, for mother's heart is
   full to the brim with love, and if you come
   to snatch only one little kiss from her no
   one will grudge it."

Rabindranath Tagore
(1861-1941)
*Translated from the Bengali
by the author*

*Reprinted with permission of Macmillan Publishing Co., Inc. from *The Crescent Moon* by Rabindranath Tagore. Copyright 1913 by Macmillan Publishing Company, Inc., renewed 1941 by Rabindranath Tagore.

RISPETTI: ON THE DEATH OF A CHILD*

I thought I heard a knock on the door.
And I jumped up as if you were here again,
Speaking to me, as you so often did,
In a coaxing tone: "Daddy, may I come in?"

When at eventide I walked along the steep seashore
I felt your small hand quite warm in mine.

And where the tide had rolled up stones,
I said aloud: "Look out that you don't fall!"

Paul Heyse
(1830-1914)
Translated from the German
by E.H. Mueller

*Reprinted from *Poetry for Pleasure, The Hallmark Book of Poetry* by permission of Hallmark Cards, Inc.

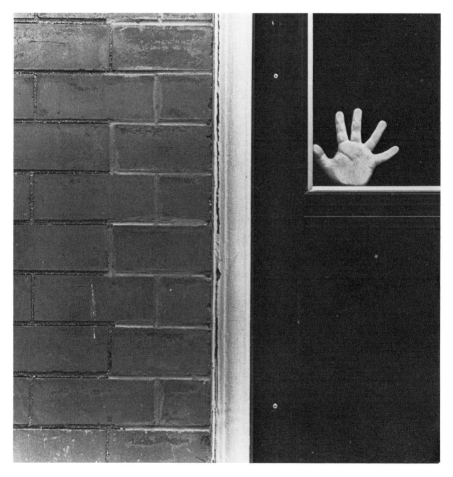

Photograph by Karen Dusenbery. (Courtesy of St. Louis Information and Counseling Program for Sudden Infant Death.)

Life goes on as it was and death is rejected. Eventually the parents may be able to allow the emptiness to occupy them and grieve for the dead child.

Parents experience this loss in every part of their being. Their bodies hurt, aching with emptiness and fatigue for which there is no rest. The parents may not be able to sleep or may find in excessive sleep an escape. Nightmares and dreams of the child are common. Patterns of concentration are interrupted. Wishes for the dead child may bring his image, his voice, his touch, his footsteps into the parent's thoughts as if the child were there. The expression of parental grief knows no bounds. The parent may even fear madness.

REACTIONS TO PARENTAL GRIEF

Families in grief for a dead child member receive inadequate recognition for the intensity and significance of their loss. There are no labels to establish the bereaved parent as someone who has experienced a significant loss. If a husband dies, the wife is called a widow; if the wife dies, the husband becomes a widower. Likewise, if a child loses the parent, the child becomes an orphan. How do we recognize the parent of a dead child?

Perhaps parents are not given recognition for the intensity of their loss because a child's death is not fully recognized as a significant loss. It is in living over years that value is attained. The value of life is weighed in terms of the number of accomplishments or quality in achievements—the more, the greater the loss. The child is not felt to have contributed much in a short life; it is even assumed that a few short years of memories are grieved faster or more completely than many long years of relating. Rather, it is the nature of the relationship and the meaning of the lost member to the survivors that is significant. Or do we deny parents their anguish because of our unwillingness to confront the intensity of such a loss? We deny and push away painful expressions. The reasons may be multiple, but the outcome predictable, that is, parents are insufficiently recognized, appreciated, and supported in their grief for their child.

Typically, bereaved families are shunned by others, who see their grief and look away. It may be that death itself is feared—so that onlookers fear contamination—that death and tragedy will spread to them and consume their happiness. Rarely will others accept the dead child's clothing or possessions for fear that death accompany them. Others want the bereaved parents to hide their agony because they are made to feel uncomfortable and their own fear of death is evoked.

Rather quickly family members learn that if they cover their feelings, they will be better received than if they show their wounds and share their feelings. As a result, a vast number of bereaved parents go underground, often unconnected even to each other. It is difficult to derive acceptance and support from others who are afraid, threatened, and unwilling to share pain.

Sharing in loss helps to validate the parent's experience and offer needed acceptance. But for many people, a sense of impotence and helplessness pervades, hampering their ability to reach out. Powerlessness takes over as onlookers try to convince themselves that they do not know how to help or what will help and therefore leave the bereaved parent with empty phrases or in solitude. They hope that the bereaved parents will get on with living, forget, and mobilize their energies to be productive again. Grieving parents may be greeted with impatience and frustration for not recovering fast enough or for continuing to remember their dead child.

Reactions to parental and family grief are varied. More often than not, parents receive inadequate recognition and support for the devastating loss that they have experienced on the death of their child.

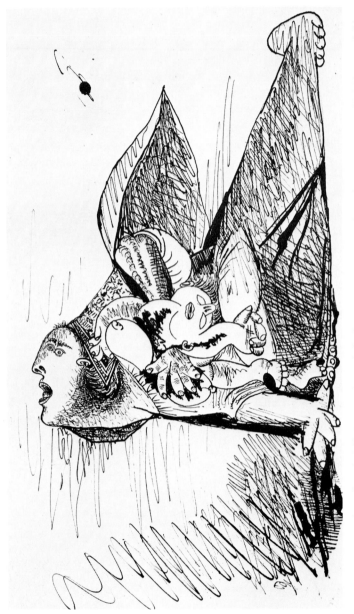

PABLO PICASSO. *Mother and Dead Child.* Composition study for *Guernica.* May 9, 1937. Ink on white paper, 9½ × 17⅞″ (On extended loan to The Museum of Modern Art, New York, from the estate of the artist.)

Suggested Readings

Fischoff, J., and O'Brien, N. After the child dies. *The Journal of Pediatrics,* January 1976, 88(1), 140-146.

Immaculate, Sr. M. (Ed.). *The cry of Rachel: An anthology of elegies on children.* New York: Random House, 1966.

Lindbergh, A.M. *Hour of gold, hour of lead: Diaries and letters of Anne Morrow Lindbergh. 1929-1932.* New York: Harcourt Brace Jovanovich, Inc., 1973.

Moffat, M.J. (Ed.). *In the midst of winter: Selections from the literature of mourning.* New York: Random House, 1982.

Parks, M.C. *Studies of grief in adult life.* New York: International Universities Press, Inc., 1972.

Sanders, C.M. A comparison of adult bereavement in the death of a spouse, child, and parent. *Omega,* 1979-80, *10*(4), 303-322.

Schiff, H.S. *The bereaved parent.* New York: Penguin Books, 1978.

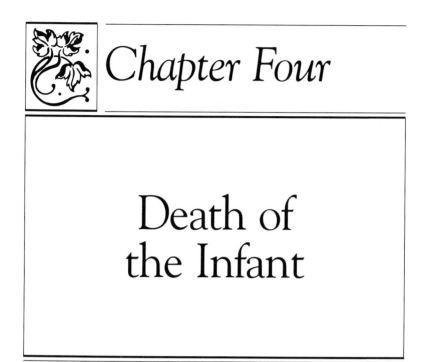

Chapter Four

Death of
the Infant

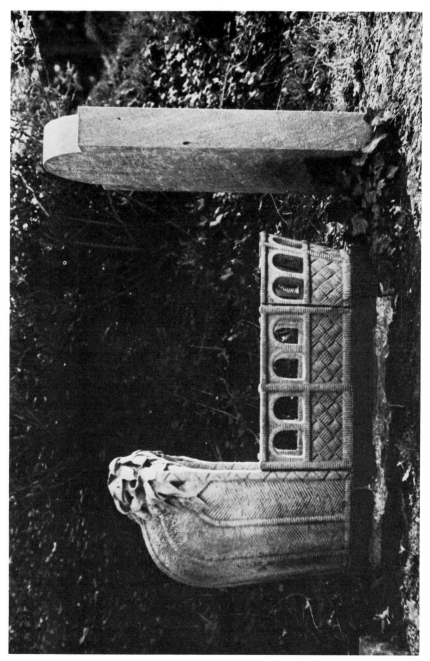

48

ON THE DEATH OF A NEW BORN CHILD*

The flowers in bud on the trees
Are pure like this dead child
The East wind will not let them last.
It will blow them into blossom.
And at last into the earth.
It is the same with this beautiful life
Which was so dear to me.
While his mother is weeping tears of blood,
Her breasts are still filling with milk.

Mei Yao Ch'en
(1002-1060)

*Kenneth Rexroth, One Hundred Poems from the Chinese. Copyright © 1971 by Kenneth Rexroth. All rights reserved. Reprinted by permission of New Directions.

THE MOST BEAUTIFUL AND MAGNIFICENT GIFT OF ALL IS LIFE itself. A baby is exactly that: new life, the antithesis of death. This new life offers boundless possibilities for loving, caring, and growing, for freshness, purity, discovery, and hope. A baby is a remarkable, sensitive, competent, and capable human being.

A baby is conceived out of intimacy and the parents' wish to join love and desire in a union of themselves. New life is created in a new form of love, more than they had shared together. A baby also comes from a desire and decision to bring into their lives, through the process of adoption, a child to become their own.

Pregnancy or the time of anticipation may be long and mysterious. Much is unknown. Much time is spent waiting. With time and growth, the new life becomes more familiar. The parents develop an attachment to their child—a person long before his arrival. The child is of them and yet a stranger to them, a new, separate, emerging self. The coming of the child is a welcome time, a time of greeting and getting to know someone long awaited. It is also a time when one's fears and fantasies are reduced or realized. Reality takes over as the parents meet their anticipated child.

A baby represents the hope for new life, new beginnings. With the dilemmas and disappointments of living, this creation is close to perfection and perhaps the only act of perfection achievable. A baby is someone to whom love can be expressed without fear, question, or reservation. Coming from us, being part of us, a baby cannot be taken away. For those who are deprived of wealth and possessions and even dignity, a baby is all of these and something that one cannot be stripped of by circumstance or external decision.

A baby represents hope for the future, hope of a better life, hope of greater opportunities, a reaching beyond. Contained in a baby are the parents' identifications that are carried within for all times. The child of our own childhood is carried through a new life. A baby represents the potential for fulfilling dreams, a way of starting over, another chance to alter the course of a lifetime. A baby is dreams and fantasies.

A baby also evokes fears and responsibilities. There is the fear that life can be snuffed out quickly, that some accident might end this dream, or that the energy will cease as disease or catastrophe surround life and consume it. The helplessness of the infant evokes in the parent an awareness of the awesome responsibility as a parent to protect the child and to sustain the life that she has created.

ONENESS OF PARENT AND CHILD

A critical feature of normal development during early infancy is the experience of oneness for parent and child. The infant remains connected to the parent and continues to be dependent on the parent for the fulfillment of his wishes and for nurture. The parent has become a person with a new identity—a parent to his child. The parent's physical and emotional sense of self is extended beyond himself and through the infant child. Parents accept this role as a commitment; they expect to provide for their child. They will give love to sustain the child and hope that, as sadness is minimized and dreams are fulfilled, this life will be better than their own.

The complex and everevolving relationship of parent to infant child is typified by many unknowns as each gets to know and love the other. The relationship is also characterized by ambivalence; the baby is welcomed and greeted with wonder and desire by the parents and yet they may feel the need for distance and reprieve as they contemplate all the changes that this baby brings. The parents lose and grieve the style of living that they knew before the child arrived.

New life is celebrated. The baby brings joy, embodies dreams and fantasies, and alerts the parents to the enormous responsibility that they have undertaken. Parents expect to see their children grow and mature. They hope to live long enough for grandchildren to be born and grow. Parents expect ultimately to die and leave their children without them but able to manage well with a direction and purpose. This is the natural course of life events; the life cycle continuing as it should. The infant then is the hope of life's new beginning. A baby is least of all expected to die.

Each infant has his own special reason for being, his own meaning to the parent. Each baby has his own special personality and place in the family with expectations for his being. The baby may signify the culmination of a loving relationship between two people or be thought of as an accident, a form of punishment, a means to establish independence, or an object to fill an empty void—or many more stated and unstated meanings. Each baby comes into a preexisting set of circumstances and relationships; each child will have his own influence in his family. The meaning that the baby carries for each member of the family will be reflected in the experience of grief and loss expressed by each member. Death strikes in the midst of the complexities of these developing relationships. Children are not always planned for and do not necessarily come at the right time with all the proper resources available.

A young woman of 15, overweight and childlike, lived with her elderly, adoptive parents. She became pregnant by a very popular schoolmate who used hallucinatory drugs regularly. She was thrilled to have been noticed and to have been loved, but she knew little about her own body and about pregnancy. She successfully concealed her pregnancy from her parents—terrified and unsure about what was happening to her body—until she delivered quite prematurely alone in her bedroom. The parents heard her cries and went to help her; they were overcome by what they found. The baby, born with

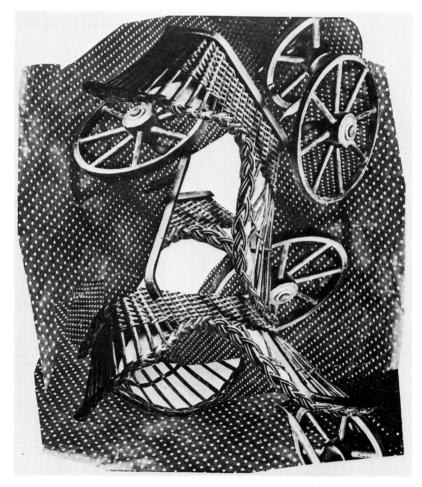

Hannah Höch. *Der Unfall.* 1936. Collage, 30.5 × 26.7 (Reprinted with permission from Marianne Carlberg-Höch, private collection.)

multiple anomalies, lived for many months in a neonatal intensive care unit until he died. The grandparents and the mother visited regularly. There was no preparation for the child, no planning, and he never lived at home. But he was deeply missed and deeply mourned.

A young mother lived alone with her baby, who suffered from heart disease and repeated episodes of protracted apnea. For the many months that he lived she held him all day long, guarding his life while she cooked and cleaned and even when she used the bathroom; she was relieved by a friend to sleep a few hours or to shower. The mother did everything that she could to keep her baby alive. When her son died, the mother's grief was overwhelming, her emptiness agonizing.

THE ULTIMATE DEPRIVATION

A baby's life holds much meaning. Making a baby may be a way of giving love or of being loved; a way of building self-esteem, of feeling proud, and of being accomplished in something; a reason for living; and a bridge to the future, to a better life. For some, living in poverty compounds the nature of life's dilemmas and offers few, if any, alternative solutions for coping. People living in poverty have little control, with few options; often a baby is all that is truly their own. A baby's death becomes the ultimate deprivation—to be stripped of all meaning; to face the senselessness of life; to be convinced there is no justice, no humanity. This is particularly poignant when one considers that many infant deaths occur in families living in poverty. For some parents this assault may epitomize their powerlessness and remind them of the deprivations and dehumanizing experiences that they have already suffered. For others, this may be their first association with death.

Regardless of circumstances, the infant's protector and nurturer is the parent. This responsibility is enormous. When an infant dies, this new sense of self and self-esteem as parent is shattered. The parent is left without a child. The infant's death leaves the parent dead inside as though the child had been ripped out of him; the emptiness that remains aches for this child. The child's space is empty. The parent continues to parent.

> This space is with me all the time it seems. Sometimes the empty space is so real I can almost touch it. I can almost see it. It gets so big sometimes that I can't see anything else. *

Many unknowingly assume that when an infant lives only a short time or dies before his birth through miscarriage, stillbirth, or abortion, the loss is not as great as the loss of an older child, who has lived longer and is more known. It may be expressed that a baby is not yet fully developed as a real person. The baby may not be perceived as a productive and contributing individual. Therefore, a baby's death is often valued less by others and by society as a whole. Somehow it is falsely assumed that not enough time had passed for the child to be missed significantly. Attachments formed with the parents and family are not recognized as deep and lasting. Less recognition is given to the child's identity and meaning to the family. This may be particularly so for the baby who is born before time or delivered dead and therefore is less tangible. However, the relationship of parent and infant is powerful; in any event a lasting attachment has been formed that endures in strength for years and years despite the length of the child's life. Parents grieve deeply for their baby and for what they will never know of him. They must also contend with the inner death that they feel.

SEARCHING TO BE WHOLE

Parents often search for ways to feel whole again when their baby dies. They yearn to feel their baby next to them—their arms full with child rather than aching to love him. The empty uterus aches. A common reaction is to suggest to parents that they have another child as if it were possible somehow to replace the lost child with a new

---

*Words by Mary Sennewald. (Courtesy of St. Louis Information and Counseling Program for Sudden Infant Death.)

one, to wipe out their pain. This attitude also implies that it is somehow easier to replace a baby than an older child, who has made more of a mark on their lives by virtue of his years of living and sharing. But this infant cannot be replaced or forgotten.

A mother was not given the opportunity to see or hold her stillborn child. She was also prevented from planning or being present for the burial of her child by a family that sought to protect her. This woman's fantasies about her child became nightmares; she searched and searched for some representation of her child. She needed desperately to identify and hold her baby, to make contact with her child and to feel whole again.

> I kept searching for something. I wasn't sure what it was. All of a sudden one day in the kitchen, I spontaneously got out my kitchen scales and started weighing fruits and vegetables. I realized I was trying to find something that had the identical weight that the baby did. . . . I found myself weighing my rolling pin . . . and it happened to be the identical length and weight that the baby was. (Davidson, 1979, pp. 12-13)

The death of an infant affects all family members and others who were attached or made some emotional investment in the baby. No one in the family is exempt from feelings of loss and grief.

Grief on the death of an infant is manifested through a wide range of normal expressions of mourning. A tremendous amount of energy is focused on planning for the child in life; when death occurs, this energy remains but is rechanneled. The energy is for parenting; these functions continue and are manifested through expressions in grief. Grieving is a process of making meaning from loss and life without the baby. The baby is a very important person with feelings and responses, whose personality and presence will be missed. The growing relationship and the joys received from the infant's capabilities are profound. His death is the ending of a sensitive, capable human life. Caring for that child cannot end with death—it continues on. Because the thought of death is so intolerable and permanent and the emptiness pervasive, the only resort is to think of the baby as alive or present in some way. The parent will continue to perform the tasks of

MATERNITY*

One wept whose only child was dead,
New-born, ten years ago.
"Weep not; he is in bliss," they said.
She answered, "Even so,

"Ten years ago was born in pain
A child, not now forlorn.
But oh, ten years ago, in vain,
A Mother, a mother was born."

Alice Meynell
(1847-1923)

*From The Poems of Alice Meynell. Courtesy of The Bodley Head, London, England.

parenting. A parent may awaken to check on the baby or buy formula or baby food. Seeing the baby or hearing the baby cry are common occurrences. Some parents wonder whether the baby is warm enough in his grave on a cold day or protected from the rain on wet days.

These experiences can be terrifying because the underlying fear is of madness. This is an expected and necessary part of the grieving process. This is shock and denial and continued attachment between parent and child. The death of one's infant is too difficult to imagine so that in a sense one returns to times when life was happier and more fulfilling, and one continues to parent by keeping the child safe. The infant was totally dependent on his parents. They gave life through love and continued it through protection and nourishment; in spite of the infant's death, the parents still seek to love and protect. Their sense of worth existed in their ability to give life; now they feel themselves dying too. Continuing to care assists in preserving their identity as worthwhile parents.

Although getting through the whole day is a most difficult task, nighttime seems especially painful. It is quiet and uninterrupted; one's thoughts are free to wander and one feels a special sense of aloneness. The aloneness can be exaggerated by relatives and friends who think that it is more therapeutic to protect the parents from their pain—and so they may refrain from speaking about the baby. Unfortunately this only makes the parents feel more alone, confused, and unable to cope with their anger and rage of being cheated. They are fearful that they will lose their baby forever because everyone is denying his existence. Denying him is like denying their own existence.

Sleep is difficult to achieve and is interrupted by nightmares—frightful images leaving one filled with remorse and fatigue. Sexuality becomes an issue. Some parents will find themselves wanting sex more often, wanting to become pregnant to fill the emptiness. Some may be terrified of another child, fearing that every child whom one loves will die, fearing sex because of the possibility of another pregnancy and more suffering. Some may feel different from the partner. Some may feel cheated and filled with hatred at the sight of another pregnant person or at families with thriving babies. Some will feel anger at the world for their injustice, anger with God for being selected for suffering, anger with the baby for dying and leaving. Comfort may be found while lying together and holding each other, asking no more of each other. This shared intimacy provides support and is a source of energy.

Photographs taken of the child while he lived and at his death compiled in an album often become a link with him. Cherishing pictures of the baby, perhaps being afraid to look at them but needing to keep them, talking with the baby and about the baby, treasuring sacred mementos left of the child: these are ways of grieving, ways of keeping connected. To keep close to the child, the parent may pin an article of clothing such as a piece of the baby's T-shirt to an undergarment. The blanket in which the baby was wrapped at the time of death may never be washed and be saved, for it continues to hold his memory and his smell. Sharing memories of the child is a way of keeping close and also helping to heal oneself. Frequent repetition of stories involving the events and circumstances of the baby's life and death become a way of reliving and keeping connected with the baby. Often the bereaved family finds that they need to take the initiative and convey the necessity of talking about the baby.

Sometimes the baby's clothes and furniture are saved to keep his memory and his presence alive. Parents may also wish to share these loved objects of their child with relatives and friends, who often find it difficult to receive, for fear that death comes with them. Some parents leave the baby's room as it was, preserving it like a shrine, and find comfort in it.

During a visit some weeks after her baby's death, a mother greeted a nurse with warmth, as if she were an old friend; yet they had never met. She began by talking about her child, from her pregnancy through his death. Her child's room was still very much alive despite his death. Brightly colored, striped sheets decorated the crib with a mobile above. His dresser was filled with his clothes; his certificate of birth was framed and in its proper place on the wall. The room was intact and much like a museum, for it preserved history, the family history. The mother was unable to put anything away. Relatives and friends had completely stopped talking about the baby—denying his existence—in their attempt to help this mother cope with her loss. She could not let go of her child and refused to give in. She was going to keep her child alive in the only way that she could; the house would remain as it was when he was alive. Further, she began to realize that if she put things away, she would be accepting his death; she had fears about her own ability to cope with her loss. She felt that she would go crazy from anguish and never stop crying once she started. It took time to work with this mother; she needed time to let down her defenses slowly and begin to feel what she had to feel to get beyond this point by expressing her grief.

Another mother described her grief this way. She said that wherever she went, she saw her child—in supermarkets, on television, in the eyes of another child, and sometimes in his carriage, where he often had taken his nap. Her own body served only to remind her that she was a parent who could not parent her child while her breasts continued to fill with milk and then later when the milk ceased.

The day's mail with coupons for diapers and baby magazines tests the parent's strength and fortitude. The world is filled with children who remind and make the empty parent feel jealous and cheated. Some parents feel a need for distance and may give away the baby's clothing, furniture, and other mementos, trying to wipe out reminders. Many parents will move to a different home, feeling that they cannot live in the same place that they lived with their child. It is often difficult to locate a family after their child's death.

Whether one searches for the child or searches for distance, there is no real peace and there are no real answers to be found for why death took the child. A baby's death is senseless. A baby is a part of his parents, less the separate person and more an extension of them. A baby is pure, perfect, amazing, and dependent, new life with new hope. A baby is part of the parents' self that can reach beyond their life and their limitations. A baby is the embodiment of their dreams and wishes, giving them a feeling of satisfaction and a sense of creativity and gratification that cannot be found in any other relationship. Each memory is important; each memory is seared to the parents' very being. The dead child will always be a baby, sweet and perfect—if only he had lived.

And can it be that in a world so full and busy,
the loss of one weak creature makes a void in any
heart, so wide and deep that nothing but the width
and depth of vast eternity can fill it up!

Charles Dickens
Dombey and Son

Reference

Davidson, G.W. *Understanding: Death of the wished-for child.* Springfield, Ill.: OGR (Order of the Golden Rule) Service Corporation, 1979. Film and pamphlet.

Suggested Readings

Borg, S., and Lasker, J. *When pregnancy fails: Families coping with miscarriage, stillborn and infant death.* Boston: Beacon Press, 1981.

Furman, E.P. The death of a newborn: Care of the parents. *Birth and the Family Journal,* Winter 1978, 5(4), 214-218.

Hagan, J.M. Infant death: Nursing interaction and intervention with grieving families. *Nursing Forum,* 1974, 13(4), 371-385.

Kennell, J., Slyter, N., and Klaus, M. The mourning response of parents to the death of a newborn infant. *New England Journal of Medicine,* 1970, 283(7), 344-349.

Kirkley-Best, E., and Kellner, K. Grief at stillbirth: An annotated bibliography. *Birth and the Family Journal,* Summer 1981, 8(2), 91-99.

Peppers, L.G., and Knapp, R.J. *Motherhood and mourning: Perinatal death.* New York: Praeger Publishers, 1980.

Schodt, C.M. Grief in adolescent mothers after an infant death. *Image,* February/March 1982, 14(1), 20-25.

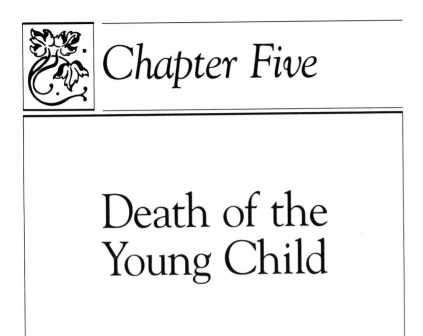

Chapter Five

Death of the Young Child

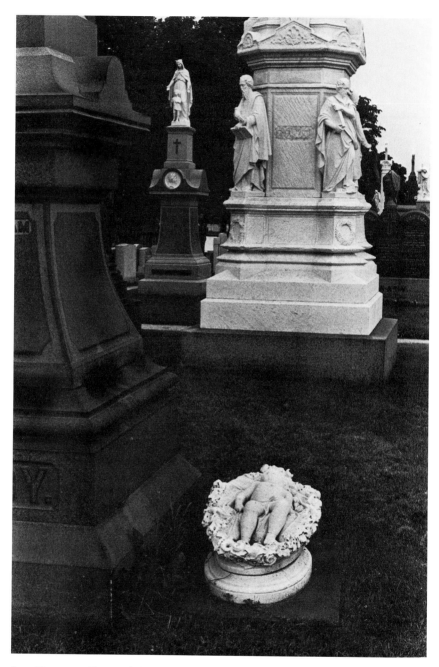

THE DEATH OF A CHILD AFTER INFANCY IS A SPECIAL AND most difficult loss for a family. This child, while connected to his parents in his dependency and vulnerability, has moved into a position in the family where he is more of a separate individual, not entirely a part of his parents. His temperamental patterns, which emerged during infancy, have been translated into his day-to-day working and playing and relating to people. As he grows, there is recognition of his talents and abilities as well as his limitations. His person is discovered as it becomes fuller and more recognizable. The parts of it that resemble or reflect parental and sibling ways are noted; the whole person containing that composite of parts that have come together in new and unique patterns is a mystery. This mystery changes from day to day as the young child grows, makes his mark on his world, and is influenced by it. The magic that we term *develop-ment* occurs within the child in the context of his family and reflects what is allowed and fostered by them.

As the young child grows, he elicits responses from his parents, siblings, other family members, and friends that range from positive to negative. There are reward and punishment, praise and correc-

A MOTHER TO HER DEAD CHILD[*]

. . . The earth: she is too old for your little body,
Too old for the small tenderness, the kissings
In the soft tendrils of your hair. The earth is so old
She can only think of darkness and sleep, forgetting
That children are restless like the small spring shadows.
But the huge pangs of winter and the pain
Of the spring's birth, the endless centuries of rain
Will not lay bare your trusting smile, your tress,
Or lay your heart bare to my heart again
In your small earthly dress. . . .

My little child who preferred the bright apple to gold,
And who lies with the shining world on his innocent eyes,
Though night-long I feel your tears, bright as the rose
In its sorrowful leaves, on my lips, and feel your hands
Touching my cheek, and wondering, "Are those your tears?"
O grief, that your heart should know the tears that seem
    empty years
And the worlds that are falling!

Edith Sitwell
(1887-1964)

[*]Reprinted from *The Collected Poems of Edith Sitwell* by permission of the publisher, Vanguard Press, Inc. Copyright © 1968, by Vanguard Press, Inc. Copyright © 1949, 1953, 1954, 1959, 1962, 1963, by Dame Edith Sitwell.

tion, which depend on his behavior and what is encouraged in the context in which he lives. He moves out in play and work into wider areas of exposure outside of his family. The young child plays with friends, attends school, begins to negotiate with other adults and children.

When the young child dies, his loss is deeply felt and mourned by his family and by the circle of important friends and acquaintances whom his life has touched. Memories of the young child are the special possession of not only parents but also teachers and friends. The important times are remembered; the store of memories can be shared and expanded upon.

Parents most often remember the child as they knew him, that is, the age at which he died. Rituals are important as the family seeks to retain a connection to the dead child. One family noted that they continued to set a place at the table for their seven-year-old child who had died. Not to do so denied the fact of the child's existence and space within the family. This same family hung and filled their child's Christmas stocking alongside that of the surviving sister. Each one in the family contributed a gift that would have been appreciated by the child now dead. The gifts given over years were for the child always seven.

Photographs of the dead child occupy a central position in the family's home. His presence is visible and all family members will relate in their own way with this child.

Clothing and possessions that are accumulated by most children, representing their movement from one season or one size to the next and from one interest or skill to another, serve as visible and concrete reminders of the child's mark on his widening world. What to do with those possessions becomes a problem for some after the child dies. Are they saved or given away? One mother gathered from her seven surviving children the special possessions—some collections and favorite toys or pieces of clothing—that reminded them of their brother. She put them away in a special box and suggested that the children rummage through the box and recall how the child used the various items. Her house rule was that this rummaging must not be done alone.

Memories of the child's contributions and favorite activities with other family members are cherished. One father noted that the house had become a source of comfort to him, for when his seven-year-old son was alive they had repaired shingles together. When he was especially lonely for his son, the father would look at the nails driven by the child and would remember the time shared.

When he dies, the young child leaves behind him large empty spaces in his family, his circle of friends, school, and community. Because the young child is fully connected to his family and occupies a special space in that system, his loss will be most keenly felt here. His person is missed as are his contributions in the form of the special tasks, responsibilities, and roles assigned to him. In addition the parents mourn their expectations of who the young child might have been, what he might have become, their wishes, hopes and dreams, developmental potential only hinted at. They also long for the love given so freely and the sparkling face filled with joy. The endless questions about how things work and why they happen, the pure reactions and responses, the thrill and excitement of new experiences and of mastery are sorely missed. Yearned for are the tears that flow freely but are redirected into smiles with the parents' touch and hugs.

Parents yearn for a return of the treasured moments, the happy times as well as the aggravations, for another opportunity to touch, see, feel the child who is gone. There are regrets for the harsh responses, the unfair expectations, the angry, negative feelings. The longing and sadness are poignantly described by a mother of a 21-month-old child who died unexpectedly. She wrote "With His Playclothes On" on the morning of her son's funeral.

The child known beyond his family is mourned by his friends, their families, and the community. The school-age child who has been involved in group activities, scouts, church groups, and clubs leaves empty spaces in all of those. Parents may find comfort in the statements of sadness and loss expressed by others who had known their child as if the child's value is confirmed and the magnitude of the loss better understood. One family from a closely knit inner-city neighborhood derived comfort from the fact that on the day of their 11-year-old's funeral service, the streets were lined with children from the school. All were dressed in white and all carried flowers. They

WITH HIS PLAYCLOTHES ON[*]

You lie there sleeping, my little son
with long dark hair
and your playclothes on.

How many times I'd pray that you'd sleep
one more hour-a day-a week,
so I could wash, or clean, or bake
a pie—some cookies—or a cake.

How many times when the house was clean
I'd get upset because you'd spill your juice
—or crumble a cookie—or drip your
bottle all over the steps.

If only you'd wake up
in my bad dream and
throw your bottle
or stand there and scream.

If only we could
see you smile—
or spill your cereal
on our new tile.

Dear God—Give me strength to forget
the bad days I had—
when I got upset
with this little lad.

With his long dark hair,
with his curls and his smiles,
who lies there sleeping
with his playclothes on.

Jay Kocheff

[*]Reprinted from *With His Playclothes On* by Dr. Glen W. Davidson by permission of OGR Service Corporation, Springfield, Illinois, © 1976. Film and pamphlet.

participated in the service, surrounding the grief-stricken parents and surviving brother. The mother in this family acknowledged that the family's grief was appreciated by this touching form of recognition and support.

The young child who dies is mourned by family, friends, and those whom his life has touched. While his connection to his family is altered by death, it continues through memories; the many reminders of clothes, pictures, and possessions; and the grieving that is shared with others who had known the child and had been touched by him.

WHEN THY MOTHER DEAR*

When your Dear Mother
Steps in through the door
And I lift my head
To meet her glance
Not on her face
At first does fall my gaze
But to that place
Nearer to the threshold
There, where your dear, little face
Would be
When you, bright with joy
Would come in with her
As before, my little daughter

When your Dear Mother
Steps in through the door
In shimmering candlelight
It always seems that you are with her
Stealing into the room behind her
As you used to.
Oh you, joyful glow of your
Father's chamber—
Alas, too soon, too quickly
snuffed out.

Friedrich Rückert
(1788-1866)
Translated from the German by
Doris Völlinger Cappadona.

Rückert wrote *Kindertotenlieder* in 1834 after losing his two youngest children in a scarlet fever epidemic. "When Thy Mother Dear" is the third song from *Kindertotenlieder* by Mahler.

*From the musical score, *Kindertotenlieder,* by Gustav Mahler. Used by permission of European Music Distributors Corporation, sole U.S. agent for Universal Edition.

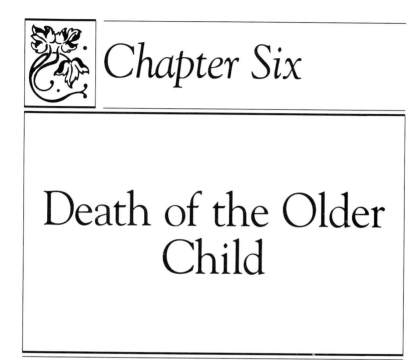

Chapter Six

Death of the Older Child

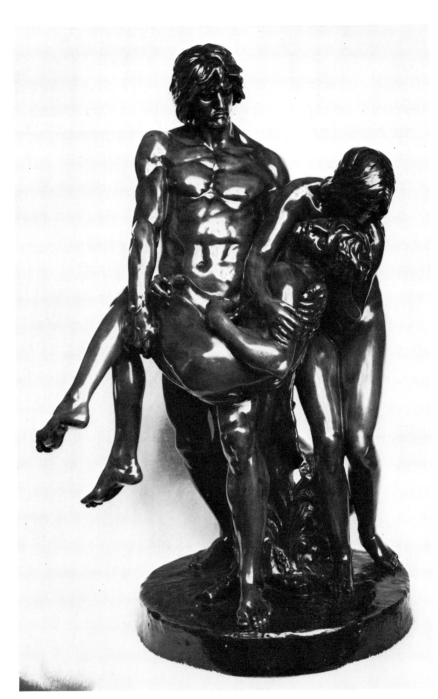

LOUIS-ERNEST BARRIOS, French, 1841-1905. *Burial of Abel.* Bronze (Collection of David Daniels, courtesy of Shepherd Gallery, New York)

THE DEATH OF AN OLDER CHILD IS A DIFFICULT AND SUBSTANtial loss to the family system. We will begin by considering adolescence and the special significance to surviving family members of child death during this critical developmental time.

THE ADOLESCENT CHILD

Adolescence is a stressful time for many young individuals and for the family systems to which they remain connected. It is a time full of unknowns and potential dangers. The years and amount of energy that many families have devoted to providing a safe, nurturing, and somewhat predictable environment are jeopardized as the adolescent moves from that setting into one that is made risky by the actual and potential dangers and by the very attitudes of the adolescent himself. Adolescence may begin chronologically at age 13 and last until the young person is 19 or entering his early 20s. Because he has lived and grown with his family over a long period of time, he is well known.

The younger the adolescent is, the more likely that he has firm connections to his family system.

As he moves into middle and late adolescence, the child will have developed relationships and connections with friends, organizations, and institutions apart from his family. Many of the struggles throughout adolescence concern the young person's move to separate from his family and to establish an identity that is uniquely his own. This developing part of the person may be strange and quite unknown to his family. As his values and modes of living change and shift away from those of his family, the adolescent clearly becomes different, more unrecognizable. His unwillingness or inability to articulate the changes that he may or may not fully understand further removes him from the communication patterns that are characteristic of his family. The changes within him, the pull to move out of his family, and the closing down of communication contribute to discord in the family.

Parental roles that were relatively sure and patterns of nurturing and caring that were manageable and effective begin to shift and change in the face of the internal and external changes in the adolescent. Parents feel less sure and less competent and angry with their adolescent for placing them in this untenable position. Where the rift is great because of the problems of adolescence and where the young person separates from his family, some parents actively mourn the loss of the child whom they knew, seeking to reconnect with him as a young adult or not at all.

Questioning their own competency, parents also fear for their adolescent as he begins to grapple with the risks, unknowns, problems, and experiences that await him. Have they as parents prepared their child well enough to do this? Is there a sturdy enough foundation laid by the family so that the adolescent can continue to grow safely and strongly? Does the adolescent possess sufficient skills, wisdom, and judgment to deal with and make decisions about peers, activities, the drugs and alcohol that are all too readily available to him. In a critical and dangerous life period where accidental injuries and suicide are the leading causes of death, parental concerns are real. The emerging adolescent with his changing moods and ways may not be sure enough of himself to impart the reassurance that his parents want most desperately to have from him.

When an adolescent child dies, a large gaping hole is left in the family fabric. The known and loved child is gone and mourned. The young person whom he was in the process of becoming is cut down. The wishes, hopes, expectations, plans of the family for this older child, whether realistic or not, are dashed by his death, never to be realized.

Responses to the Death

The anger by parents at decisions made by the adolescent, which may or may not have contributed to his death, can be enormous. There may be great guilt on the part of parents for the feelings and exchanges preceding the child's death. Parents may idealize their adolescent, remembering selectively the qualities and characteristics that they considered to be most valuable.

The adolescent, because of the need to reach out to others not in the family, has developed ties and connections to other individuals and groups. The fact that the adolescent's death is felt and mourned by others outside the family can be comforting to surviving members. The valuing of their grown child by others affirms the magnitude and importance of the loss to the family. One mother commented that she had no idea that her 13-year-old son, who recently and unexpectedly died, was so sensitive to other people. To her he appeared self-centered and absorbed in his own interests and activities while at home. This mother learned through classmates and friends that her son actively sought ways to be available to others. She felt proud and comforted by this information about her son, provided by persons who had known him apart from his family.

Families of adolescents who die may feel less responsibility for the actual cause of death if they have allowed their adolescent child some part in his own decision making. However, allowing this more active participation then may be questioned. Were they not protective enough? Could they have prevented the death had they exercised more parental control over the child and circumstances? Indeed,

The Holmes Children Stone. 1795, East Glastonbury, Connecticut, Red Sandstone, 48 × 45 (From *Graven Images: New England Stone Carving and its Symbols, 1650-1815,* by Allan I. Ludwig, Wesleyan University Press. Reprinted with permission of Allan I. Ludwig.)

part of the family growing with the adolescent child is allowing him to assume more responsibility for his actions, choices, successes, and failures. Without this gradually increasing freedom to separate, the adolescent cannot develop the autonomy that contributes to wholeness as a human being.

Parents are often left to struggle with their own guilt and enormous sense of responsibility while they find comfort in their ability to let go. One family sanctioned the decision of their only son, a 17-year-old college freshman, to hitchhike home for a holiday time. The boy was killed on the road by an erratic driver; his heartbroken parents struggled with their support of his decision and the outcome. They felt entirely responsible for his death until they recalled with the assistance of their clergy that they had vehemently opposed his decision but had not stood in his way of making it. There was small relief in sharing that enormous burden.

The adolescent with all his skills and talents and special interests leaves behind him the possessions that represent growth and change over a brief lifetime. In many homes, in every room there are visible reminders of the adolescent who filled so much space. There are items of clothing, pieces of sports equipment, books, pictures, and other belongings that mark his having been there.

In his wake are left the scores of memories of him as an infant, a young child, a child of middle years. Photographs, trophies, toys, projects remain as poignant reminders of so many years of life. They haunt and comfort the remaining family members.

More is known of the adolescent because of the time that he has spent within the family system. His strengths and limitations, his skills and weaknesses, his hopes and disappointments are known as he has shared them and are remembered in vivid detail.

Parents are left with the sense of unfairness, the bitter disappointment that they have been deprived of knowing their child as an adult, as that person separate from themselves, yet a part of them and their link to the future. Some parents believe that just as they have been deprived of knowing and watching this young person's growth to adulthood, the world is poorer for his absence.

Parental grief is tinged with the bitterness of deprivation. Having invested so much in the life of an adolescent, to have their child taken from them is devastating. Parents are helpless, impotent to intervene, and angry. Death can take the adolescent expectedly or unexpectedly and sometimes violently, aborting the natural process of separation and individuation that is healthy and characteristic for this period.

If only the parents had done more to love, to protect, to fend off death.

A Word From Frances*

Death always brings one suddenly face to face with life. Nothing, not even the birth of one's child, brings one so close to life as his death.

Johnny lay dying of a brain tumor for fifteen months. He was in his seventeenth year. I never kissed him good night without wondering whether I should see him alive in the morning. I greeted him each morning as though he were newly born to me, a re-gift of God. Each day he lived was a blessed day of grace.

The impending death of one's child raises many questions in one's mind and heart and soul. It raises all the infinite questions, each answer ending in another question. What is the meaning of life? What are the relations between things: life and death? the individual and the family? the family and society? marriage and divorce? the individual and the state? medicine and research? science and politics and religion? man, men, and God?

All these questions came up in one way or another, and Johnny and I talked about them, in one way or another, as he was dying for fifteen months. He wasn't just dying, of course. He was living and dying and being reborn all at the same time each day. How we loved each day. "It's been another wonderful day, Mother!" he'd say, as I knelt to kiss him good night.

There are many complex and erudite answers to all these questions, which men have thought about for many thousands of years, and about which they have written many thousands of books.

*Reprinted by permission of Harper & Row, Publishers, Inc. Abridged from "A Word from Frances" in *Death Be Not Proud: A Memoir* by John Gunther. Copyright, 1949, by John Gunther.

Yet at the end of them all, when one has put away all the books, and all the words, when one is alone with oneself, when one is alone with God, what is left in one's heart? Just this:

I wish we had loved Johnny more.

Since Johnny's death, we have received many letters from many kind friends from all parts of the world, each expressing his condolence in his own way. But through most of them has run a single theme: sympathy with us in facing a mysterious stroke of God's will that seemed inexplicable, unjustifiable and yet, being God's will, must also be part of some great plan beyond our mortal ken, perhaps sparing him or us greater pain or loss.

Actually, in the experience of losing one's child in death, I have found that other factors were involved.

I did not for one thing feel that God had personally singled out either him or us for any special act, either of animosity or generosity. In a way I did not feel that God was personally involved at all. I have all my life had a spontaneous, instinctive sense of the reality of God, in faith, beyond ordinary belief. I have always prayed to God and talked things over with Him, in church and out of church, when perplexed, or very sad, or also very happy. During Johnny's long illness, I prayed continually to God, naturally. God was always there. He sat beside us during the doctors' consultations, as we waited the long vigils outside the operating room, as we rejoiced in the miracle of a brief recovery, as we agonized when hope ebbed away, and the doctors confessed there was no longer anything they could do. They were helpless, and we were helpless, and in His way, God, standing by us in our hour of need, God in His infinite wisdom and mercy and loving kindness, God in all His omnipotence, was helpless too.

Life is a myriad series of mutations, chemical, physical, spiritual. The same infinitely intricate, yet profoundly simple, law of life that produced Johnny—his rare and precious soul, his sweetness, his gaiety, his gallantry, his courage: for it was only after his death, from his brief simple diaries, written as directly as he wrote out his beloved chemical experiments, that we learned he had known all along how grave was his illness, and that even as we had gaily pretended with him that all was well and he was completely recovering, he was pretending with us, and bearing our burden with the spirit, the élan, of a singing soldier or a laughing saint—that law of life which out of infinite mutation had produced Johnny, that law still mutating, destroyed him. God Himself, no less than us, is part of that law.

Johnny was an extraordinarily lovable and alive human being. There seemed to be no evil, only an illuminating good, in him. Everybody who knew him, his friends and teachers at Lincoln, Riverdale, and Deerfield, our neighbors in the country at Madison, felt the warmth of his goodness and its great vitality in him. Yet a single cell, mutating experimentally, killed him. But the law of mutations, in its various forms, is the law of the universe. It is impersonal, inevitable. Grief cannot be concerned with it. At least, mine could not.

My grief, I find, is not desolation or rebellion at universal law or deity. I find grief to be much simpler and sadder. Contemplating the Eternal Deity and His Universal Laws leaves me grave but dry-eyed. But a sunny fast wind along the Sound, good sailing weather, a new light boat, will shake me to tears: how Johnny would have loved this boat, this wind, this sunny day!

All the things he loved tear at my heart because he is no longer here on earth to enjoy them. All the things he loved! An open fire with a broiling steak, a pancake tossed in the air, fresh nectarines, black-red cherries—the science columns in the papers and magazines, the fascinating new technical developments—the Berkshire music festival coming in over the air, as we lay in the moonlight on our wide open beach, listening—how he loved all these! For like many children of our contemporary renaissance, he was many-sided, with many loves. Chemistry and math were his particular passion, but as a younger child at school, he had painted gay spirited pictures of sailing boats and circuses, had sculpted some lovable figures, two bears dancing, a cellist playing, and had played some musical instruments himself, piano, violin, and his beloved recorder. He collected stamps, of course, and also rocks; he really loved and knew his rocks, classified them, also cut and polished them in his workshop, and dug lovely bits of garnet from the Connecticut hillsides.

But the thing closest to his heart was his Chem Lab which he cherished passionately. It grew and expanded in town and country. He wanted to try experiments that had not been done before. He liked to consider abstract principles of the sciences, searched intuitively for unifying theories.

He had many worthy ambitions which he did not live long enough to achieve. But he did achieve one: graduation with his class at Deerfield. Despite the long illness that kept him out of school a year and a half, he insisted on being tutored in the hospital and at home, taking his class exams, and the college board exams for Harvard, and then returning to Deerfield for commencement week. The boys cheered him as he walked down the aisle to receive his diploma, his head bandaged but held high, his young face pale, his dark blue eyes shining with the joy of achievement. A fortnight later, he died.

What is the grief that tears me now?

No fear of death or any hereafter. During our last summer at Madison, I would write in my diary when I couldn't sleep. "Look Death in the face. To look Death in the face, and not be afraid. To be friendly to Death as to Life. Death as a part of Life, like Birth. Not the final part. I have no sense of finality about Death. Only the final scene in a single act of a play that goes on forever. Look Death in the face: it's a friendly face, a kindly face, sad, reluctant, knowing it is not welcome but having to play its part when its cue is called, perhaps trying to say, 'Come, it won't be too bad, don't be afraid, I understand how you feel, but come—there may be other miracles!' No fear of Death, no fight against Death, no enmity toward Death, friendship with Death as with Life. That is—Death for myself, but not for Johnny, God, not yet. He's too young to miss all the other parts of Life, all the other lovely living parts of life. All the wonderful, miraculous things to do, to feel, to see, to hear, to touch, to smell, to taste, to experience, to enjoy. What a joy Life is. Why does no one talk of the joy of Life? shout, sing, write of the joy of Life? Looking for books to read with Johnny, and all of them, sad, bitter, full of fear, hate, death, destruction, damnation, or at best resignation. No great books of enjoyment, no sense of great utter simple delight pleasure fun sport joy of Life."

All the things Johnny enjoyed at home and at school, with his friends, with me. All the simple things, the eating, drinking, sleeping, waking up. We cooked, we experimented with variations on pancakes, stews, steaks. We gardened, we fished, we sailed. We danced, sang, played. We repaired things, electric wires, garden tools, chopped wood, made fires. We equipped the Chem Lab Workshop, in the made-over old boathouse, with wonderful gadgets, and tried out experiments, both simple and fantastic.

All the books we read. All the lovely old children's books, and boys' books, and then the older ones. We read Shaw aloud—how G.B.S. would have enjoyed hearing the delighted laughter of the boys reading parts in *Man and Superman* in the kitchen while I washed up the supper dishes—and Plato's *Republic* in Richards' *Basic English*, and Russell, and St. Exupéry. On Sundays, we would have church at home: we'd sit outdoors on the beach and read from The Bible of the World, the Old Testament and the New, the Prophets and Jesus, also Buddha, Confucious, and Mahomet. Also Spinoza, Einstein, Whitehead, Jeans, Schroedinger, and Maugham.

We talked about everything, sense and nonsense. We talked about the news and history, especially American History, and its many varied strains; about the roots of his own great double heritage, German and Hebrew; about empires past and present, India's non-violent fight for freedom, and about reconciliation between Arabs and Jews in Palestine. We talked about Freud and the Oedipus complex, and behavior patterns in people and societies, getting down to local brass tacks. And we also played nonsense games, stunts, and card tricks.

We sailed, and got becalmed, and got tossed out to sea, and had to be rescued. And we planned sailing trips.

All the things we planned! College, and work, and love and marriage, and a good life in a good society.

We always discussed things a little ahead. In a way I was experimenting with Johnny as he dreamed of doing with his elements, as artists do with their natural materials. I was trying to create of him a newer kind of human being: an aware person, without fear, and with love: a sound individual, adequate to life anywhere on earth, and loving life everywhere and always. We would talk about all this as our experiment together.

He did his part in making our experiment a success. Missing him now, I am haunted by my own shortcomings, how often I failed him. I think every parent must have a sense of failure, even of sin, merely in remaining alive after the death of a child. One feels that it is not right to live when one's child has died, that one should somehow have found the way to give one's life to save his life. Failing there, one's failures during his too brief life seem all the harder to bear and forgive. How often I wish I had not sent him away to school when he was still so young that he wanted to remain at home in his own room, with his own things and his own parents. How I wish we had maintained the marriage that created the home he loved so much. How I wish we had been able before he died to fulfill his last heart's desires: the talk with Professor Einstein, the visit to Harvard Yard, the dance with his friend Mary.

These desires seem so simple. How wonderful they would have been to him. All the wonderful things in life are so simple that one is not aware of their wonder until they are beyond touch. Never have I felt the wonder and beauty and joy of life so keenly as now in my grief that Johnny is not here to enjoy them.

Today, when I see parents impatient or tired or bored with their children, I wish I could say to them, But they are alive, think of the wonder of that! They may be a care and a burden, but think, they are alive! You can touch them—what a miracle! You don't have to hold back sudden tears when you see just a headline about the Yale-Harvard game because you know your boy will never see the Yale-Harvard game, never see the house in Paris he was born in, never bring home his girl, and you will not hand down your jewels to his bride and will have no grandchildren to play with and spoil. Your sons and daughters are alive. Think of that—not dead but alive! Exult and sing.

All parents who have lost a child will feel what I mean. Others, luckily, cannot. But I hope they will embrace them with a little added rapture and a keener awareness of joy.

I wish we had loved Johnny more when he was alive. Of course we loved Johnny very much. Johnny knew that. Everybody knew it. Loving Johnny more. What does it mean? What can it mean, now?

Parents all over the earth who lost sons in the war have felt this kind of question, and sought an answer. To me, it means loving life more, being more aware of life, of one's fellow human beings, of the earth.

It means obliterating, in a curious but real way, the ideas of evil and hate and the enemy, and transmuting them, with the alchemy of suffering, into ideas of clarity and charity.

It means caring more and more about other people, at home and abroad, all over the earth. It means caring more about God.

I hope we can love Johnny more and more till we too die, and leave behind us, as he did, the love of love, the love of life.

—Frances Gunther

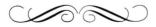

THE ADULT CHILD

While we have focused on child death spanning the period of infancy through adolescence, the family's process of grieving and living without occurs regardless of the age of the child member at death. Just as the family mourns the infant, the young child, and the adolescent, so does it mourn the adult child of any age.

The parents mourn the loss of their child, that part of themselves, the separate person and his contributions to the family life. For elderly parents who no doubt have known other losses, being predeceased by a child is intolerable and unnatural and produces a special sense of responsibility and guilt. Somehow the order of the elderly dying and the young living is disrupted and turned around. To have not intervened effectively to protect the adult child from his untimely death speaks of failure to the parent in this most important area of responsibility.

How connected that adult child is to his family of origin surely influences the responses of parents and surviving siblings. How much a part of the continuing life of that family that adult member is influences the way in which members grieve his loss.

Parents of the adult child in their process of grieving may attempt to search out clues and reasons for the death, looking back as far as conception, pregnancy, circumstances surrounding the birth, continuing through the crisis and experiences of childhood and adolescence and young adulthood. The process is longer and more difficult because of all the years that their child lived. Distortions appear in the form of rationalization and idealization; there are gaps in memory. Were there problems that parents missed? In retrospect, were they to blame for something they did not see or do?

For the parent who has become dependent on the adult child for emotional support, financial assistance, and everyday care, that child's untimely death produces hardship, deprivation, and change. Parental grief is tinged with anger and disappointment. To have been left to fend for themselves, assisted only by friends or agencies, after a period of dependency on adult offspring is a bitter and difficult reversal indeed. Who will take care of them? Who will understand them as did their own child? Will they be responsible for the care of grandchildren, a difficult task at a time when their own children have grown and died?

Parents may blame the adult child or the surviving spouse and family for not providing adequate care that they as protectors had all of their child's life with them. In addition to blame, anger for the offspring dying may be displaced onto the surviving spouse or grandchildren, causing a rift between themselves and those close to them. If the rift is great, changes in the availability of grandchildren to grandparents may represent another loss. The spouse and children may relocate to a distant area so that the normal visiting patterns are changed and contact severed with grandparents, compounding the loss sustained through death. Sorting out the questions and problems with the will or in the absence of such a statement may contribute to disputes among surviving family members.

Parents of an adult child who has died receive little recognition and sympathy while the spouse and children are the recipients of condolences and comfort. Cards, messages of support, phone calls are for the most part directed to the widows, widowers, and surviving children while parents receive little that recognizes their grief and offers solace. Indeed professional interest and study and the resultant substantial body of literature that deals with bereavement are directed to the surviving spouse or children whose parents have died.

Little has been written of parental grief for the dead child of any age. However, grief for one's young, adolescent, and adult child knows no limit.

And you watch with serenity through the winters of your grief

—Kahlil Gibran[*]

[*]Reprinted from *The Prophet*, by Kahlil Gibran, by permission of Alfred A. Knopf, Inc. Copyright 1923 by Kahlil Gibran and renewed 1951 by Administrators C.T.A. of Kahlil Gibran Estate, and Mary G. Gibran.

Suggested Readings

Agee, J. *A death in the family.* New York: Bantam Books, 1972.

Furman, E. *Studies in childhood bereavement.* New Haven: Yale University Press, 1974.

Krementz, J. *How it feels when a parent dies.* New York: Alfred A. Knopf, 1981.

Leshan, E. *Learning to say goodby when a parent dies.* New York: Macmillan, 1976.

Chapter Seven

Living Without

ON THE DEATH OF A ONLY SON

1
Here drooping by thy lifeless side,
Pensive, retir'd, with grief o'erborne!
Lovely in death my darling pride,
Thee the long weeping Muse shall mourn.

2
Farewell! thou dearest in my heart,
Whom neither tears nor prayers could save:
'Tis death's redoubled pain to part,
And leave such beauty in the grave.

3
Strong was thy wisdom wondrous, child!
Active and bright its early ray.
Thy temper grateful winning mild,
And love rul'd all the smiling day.

4
Ah me! that once such sweetness grac'd,
Those winning smiles that angel form,
Corruption's greedy train shall waste
The mould'ring dust the feasting worm.

5
By night my eyes the search repeat,
Sad to the glittering skies they roll,
Tell me, I say the happy fate,
Say where resides the blissful soul.

6
That day shall bring thee to my sight,
Thy presence shall my joys restore,
Fill me thou thought with vast delight
When death shall never part us more.

Sarah Steen's Work in the 10 year of her age

18   06

On the Death of A (sic) Only Son. Linen Sampler, American, 20½ × 12½", 1806. William B. Thayer Memorial Collection. (Courtesy of Helen Foresman Spencer Museum of Art, The University of Kansas, Lawrence, Kansas)

On the Death of an Only Son

1

Here drooping by thy lifeless side
Pensive, retir'd, with grief o'erborne
Lovely in death my darling pride,
Thee, the long weeping Muse shall mourn.

2

Farewell thou dearest in my heart,
Whom neither tears nor prayers could save:
Tis death's redoubled pain to part.
And leave such beauty in the grave.

3

Strong was thy wisdom wondrous child
Active and bright its early ray
Thy temper grateful, winning mild,
And love rul'd all the smiling day.

4

Ah me: that once such sweetness graced
Those winning smiles that angel form
Corruption's greedy train shall waste
The mouldering dust the feasting worm.

5

By night my eyes the search repeat
Sad to the glittering skies they roll
Tell me, I say the happy fate
Say where resides the blissful soul.

6

That day shall bring thee to my sight
Thy presence shall my joys restore
Fill me thou thought with vast delight
When death shall never part us more.

. . . death eventually separates everyone from each other. It is only the vividness of memory that keeps the dead alive forever.

—John Irving
The World According to Garp

GRIEVING IS A PROCESS IN WHICH WE ENGAGE IN ORDER TO cope with loss and death and to learn to live without. When the child dies, the parents learn to live without this child, yet always living with the knowledge and sensation of being "the parents of a child who has died." As survivors they are left to deal with their loss by living with pain and emptiness, aloneness and anger, and ultimately, by investing their energies in relationships with others and establishing new ties with the world. After their child's death parents may wonder if it is truly possible to live without this child. Others do, but how? If there were only something to give or sacrifice for the return of their child's life, how willingly that would be done. Parents think about their own death, perhaps to rejoin their child and be together. Physically the parents live, yet death seems to occupy them. It is as though the exterior relates and responds, perhaps happily, yet tears are shed within. The shattered survivor may move slowly, floating, drifting, apart from the outside world. Parents do not "get over" such a death. Living is learning to survive without their child. The grieving process is long—life long.

Thoughts of a Mother*
by Carolyn Szybist

I am the parent of a child who has died. The real significance of that fact is that it took me so long to come to terms with the ultimate reality of it, to accept that which is true. You don't get over the loss of a child. You don't replace him. Grief will surface unexpectedly, softer at the edges with the passage of time, but grief nonetheless. Like many of the components of each of our lives, the death of a child is something that finally you incorporate into yourself. Instead of waking up one morning being healed from your grief, you learn to live with it.

There is no easy way to lose a child. There is no disease or event that is preferable, and no age or point in time that makes a difference. Although parents who lose children may frequently empathize with others and say things like, "I'm glad that didn't happen to me," we usually mean, "I'm glad that didn't happen to me in addition to what did." As time passes, we feel an almost universal kinship with anyone who has lost a child and have a strong sense that of all our grief experiences, the death of a child is the most difficult. We all have the conception that in the scheme of things, parents are *not* supposed to outlive their children.

I am a different person from the young woman I was just before my child died. I don't feel changed in a radical sense, but I am changed. It's sometimes difficult to relate to that person: to the youth, invincibility, and near simplicity. Sometimes I have difficulty remembering that young woman who was the mother of two children, a daughter nearly 2 and a son aged 3 months, a person who could resent the moments when everybody was cranky and hungry at once and sleep seemed a remote experience, and a person who also reveled in the joys and experiences of motherhood. Tucked into those days were the joys and strains of a young marriage as my husband and I adapted and attempted to grow: the children and the two of us, completing educational goals and beginning professional careers. It was a good time, laced with all the happiness and minor dissensions that are part of living.

*Reprinted with permission from Sahler, Olle Jane Z., editor: *The child and death*, St. Louis, 1978, The C.V. Mosby Co. and with permission from the author and editor.

And in one hellish moment, all of that changed. Changed as swiftly as if a bomb had been dropped into the core of our lives. Changed on a bright, sunny summer morning when I picked up the rigid, lifeless, distorted body of our young son. Changed as swiftly as he must have died. Part of the hell was the fact that his death was not expected. Part of the hell was the fact that the year was 1965 and his death from crib death was a phenomenon not well understood, especially by me, his mother, who as a nurse took pride in some knowledge of disease. Most of the hell came simply from the fact that he was dead and from all the events that followed because he was dead.

I'm grateful for the haziness that enveloped me from the beginning of that terrible moment. The attempts by my husband to resuscitate the tiny little body, and my own rejection of the deadness of him. After that first moment of discovery, my inability to touch him. The horrendous anger of my husband (that was shared with me later), that while he tried to revive our son, what he wanted to do was hurl his body across the room as if to deny that the cold body could have ever held the personality of his son. The silly decisions that come with what to do with the young daughter, confined to her own crib, who is baffled by the madness of her parents. The wild dash to the hospital emergency room, the irrevocable pronouncement of death, the shared disbelief of the physician who had brought this child into the world and cared for him in those early days. The convergence of relatives from across the country interspersed with autopsy reports and questions, asked and unasked. The image of the distorted face of my son's body from the mottled blueness of death, an image eased somewhat by the dressed and made-up body in the tiny white casket. And the pain that came from deep inside my chest and radiated relentlessly to every part of my body. The inability to eat or sleep, and the insane ability to talk to people about things I didn't care about. I know I smiled at the funeral, thanked people for coming, laughed about the population explosion that we would participate in, as if another baby would make things right. I also know that I wasn't really there. I performed as carefully as a well-rehearsed script, except that the performance was staged in unreality, done to ease the pain of others but done mostly because it really wasn't happening and tomorrow I could wake up to my two children and only think of the nightmare I must be dreaming.

The first twinges of reality came the evening of his funeral, came with the onset of a thunderstorm and the realness that my son was out in the rain, sleeping in a small grave among other children. I had never left a child in the rain before and the franticness of that reality was a reality in itself. The haziness was comfort; reality was sheer terror.

There is discomfort in looking back and remembering the endless days that followed the funeral. The discomfort comes from the human desire to acknowledge the fragility of others, but not of ourselves. They were days that passed for living. And days when other events were irrevocably locked into the kind of living that we did. The sudden death of my husband's 22-year-old male cousin from unclear causes came 3 weeks after my son's death. The fact that we shared the same last name brought with it my own thoughts that we were locked into a bizarre twist of fate where all the members of our family would die. I checked sleeping people in our household with the regularity of an intensive care facility and felt singularly responsible for their ability to breathe.

I became the perfect, overprotective, smothering, all-consuming parent to my young daughter. I was afraid to let her from my sight but also afraid to accept the responsibility for her care. It was a time of decisionless decisions. I was her constant companion and playmate. I needed others to help with her care, but resented their helpfulness. I marvel that either of us survived those early months when her life was changed from the patterns that she knew. And again the jolts of reality among the haze. The jolt that came with the Christmas that followed the foggy months of summer and fall and the present to my daughter, gaily wrapped and delivered with affection by a caring relative. A present torn from its wrappings with the toddler fingers to discover under the lid of the box a life-size baby doll. A present greeted with screams of pain and attempts to cover and rewrap it with the shreds of paper. And the attempts to hide from her sight what jolted us all: the return of the baby brother whose swift departure had never been acknowledged or shared with her. The sobs that finally resulted in sleep said much about our own denial that our child had died.

Denial comes in many ways. It sits beneath the surface of our statements of truth. I wanted another baby, and I was terrified of having one. It disrupted my relationship with my husband in many subtle ways. We talked, but we didn't talk. We shared, but we didn't share. He was alternately strong and compassionate and angry and unfeeling. And sometimes we hated each other and ourselves, but never openly. Our sex life was mostly bad. Tenderness and need can get lost in fear of pregnancy and fear of being incapable of good parenting. And just fear in general.

When I look back, one word describes it best of all. Lonely. No matter what the activity, or how many people were around, it was a lonely, vacant time. And disruptive to our total sense of living. I like to think that we did a good job of covering up our feelings, that on the surface we performed normally. It was the feelings just under the surface of that cover that were either astir or just an enormous void. It was hard to talk to anyone about that baby. A mention of even good times involving him could bring a conversation to an uncomfortable standstill.

There were moments when I began to search relentlessly through the medical literature and libraries for information about crib death. And days when I believed that he had died of the interstitial pneumonitis that appeared on the all-knowing death certificate. Those were the days that I knew I must be a terrible mother and obviously a lousy nurse. Pneumonia was curable. But not for my child and probably because of me. No one ever really accused me, but frequently I accused myself. And there were days when I couldn't bear to hear about him at all, much less any speculation of why he died. The very mention of the word dead or death in the lightest of conversation sent sensations of pain all the way to my toes.

The pregnancy in the following spring that resulted in a miscarriage was probably the lowest point of all. The pain was real, and this time there was really no one to share that with, or so it seemed. The death of that son was a closed book. And the months that followed were as sterile as my inability to become pregnant again.

When do you start to "get better?" The landmarks don't exist until you can get far enough away to start to look back at them. And landmarks are really events that you are finally ready for. For me, there was the article in a woman's magazine about crib death. An article I read exactly 3 years after the death of my son. I had read other articles, but this one sparked something inside of me. Perhaps I was ready for what it had to say. That article somehow led me to a list of names of other people, who in turn were given my name. In one overwhelming week, I found myself talking on the telephone to 14 other parents. For each of us it was the first time we had ever really talked to anyone "like" us. And the release inside of me of so many locked up feelings can only be described as nearly exhilarating. It was a strange blend of hearing other people say what I had been feeling, and feeling along with them what I was hearing them say. When we all finally met as a group, it can only be described as a warm reunion of very old friends; there were no strangers.

To "get involved" with other parents was a landmark in itself. The majority of my relatives and friends, particularly my health professional friends, were concerned and fearful that this kind of activity could only be destructive—especially 3 years later. How could I go about the business of forgetting, which I should have already done, and at the same time associate with families who had lost children? That landmark took on new meaning that I was much slower to perceive. The quiet, strong support for what was happening to me came from an unexpected, and yet should have been expected, source: my husband. The sharing that wasn't his need was acknowledged by him as being mine, and the real encouragement to "be involved" came from him. It sometimes baffles his children to this day that he doesn't talk much about that young son, but I know he feels. We all work out our greatest pains in our own ways, and there is no right or wrong for each of us. Just different ways. Grief is staggeringly self-centered. I sometimes feel a sense of sadness for the too many lonely days that might not have all had to be if we had known that simple truth, if someone had pointed out that those differences don't have to isolate you from each other. I'm only grateful that somehow we learned it.

To "be involved" with other parents and crib death in the 1960s was an experience of its own. The groups became islands for others like us in a world that knew very little about us. I never made a conscious decision to get involved in crib death as a cause. As with so many others like me across the country, it is better explained by saying that it happened by simply happening—whatever our needs or reasons.

At the very beginnings of my involvement with other parents came the long-awaited pregnancy and the arrival of another son. The baby, like the group involvement, was blessing and disruption, joyful and fearful, good and bad. Sometimes we worried about the baby. Other times we accepted that if he died, too, it might be beyond our control. There were moments when the awareness of crib death loomed over our heads, and that awareness was resented. There were more times when that knowledge was a comfort. And there were days when it was important to hide from the fact that other children were dying. And days when we could face that fact without discomfort. We survived our son's infancy, as did he, in a period of time that was its own landmark.

In the years that followed, I am fascinated by remembering the new kind of denial that took place, a denial that I have learned to accept with some semblance of amusement at myself. There were periods of time when I wanted to believe, like so many other people, that grief has a beginning and an end. That anything less than that might require acknowledging some human instability. There were times when I questioned how anyone could be involved in a cause that had claimed the life of their child without being somewhat strange, if not actually bordering on the mentally unhealthy. Being identified as a SIDS parent meant being less than credible, and perhaps the only objective individuals were those who had never touched on the grief experiences of life. So although I could talk about my son, I often considered that he was a closed chapter of my life, that he had been loved and mourned but that was finished.

Just as I now know that the brief life of the son who died has taught me much about myself and living, I also know that it took my living son to show me a great deal about death and accepting grief. It was the most important landmark for me, and I learned it from a 6-year-old on a cold, snowy day just before Christmas 2 years ago. I hadn't planned to drive down the street I had chosen, nor had I planned on the snow or the two bickering children jailed with an intolerant mother in a car doing last-minute holiday shopping. But that street and that day took us past the cemetery where a small marker is a reminder of that child that was. The announcement by my daughter that we were passing the cemetery was almost one of retaliation to her brother, an attempt to even the score of the backseat hostilities with some special knowledge. And the announcement brought silence, a silence that was broken by the sudden demand of my son to stop, to turn into the cemetery and to see his brother. It was a turn that I made with reluctance; we so rarely stopped there anymore. It was not where I wanted to be, but I went along with his request. But it wasn't enough to trudge through the snow and locate the tiny grave. He had asked to see his brother, and he wanted to do just that. To see him, to touch him. And I knew, just as suddenly as the demand had been made, that there was some new realization present, some new significance to this brother who had been mentioned but didn't live with us. When it was finally clear that we couldn't see the body, a series of relentless questions began that were almost beyond the youngness of his mind.

"Why did he die?" "What did you do?" "Why couldn't you save him?" "What is this disease?" "Are you sure?" "Why couldn't anyone save him?" "Why my brother?" "Why me?"

And there they were, so many years later. All my questions coming back to haunt me. All the questions of any parent who has ever lost a child. And the snow became mixed with tears, mine and his, as we stood there. I cried for him, that young son caught in unexpected grief for a brother he never knew and would never know. And I cried for the daughter who somehow survived our inadequacies. And I cried for that child who would never grow up. And I cried for me. I cried with the clear knowledge that it was okay to cry, that remembering is not abnormal or strange, that there is a time and a place for remembering, that you don't ever really forget, that you learn to live with it.

I am many things. And among those things is the acceptance of an inescapable truth. I am the parent of a child who has died.

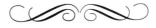

Anne Morrow Lindbergh writes: "Contrary to the general assumption, the first days of grief are not the worst. The immediate reaction is usually shock and numbing disbelief. One has undergone an amputation" (Lindbergh, 1973, pp. 212-213). Grieving is a lifelong process of learning to manage and negotiate in life without this vital part of oneself, which cannot be replaced. The raw wound may heal in some fashion, but the scar and emptiness of missing a vital person, a vital part of self and family, remain. The parents are changed; their relationship and the family constellation and interactions are altered by the child's death. Love and attachment do not die and are not limited by time. In the years that follow their child's death, parents will grieve for what was and what will never be. They will grieve their emptiness. A child's death is unacceptable. How can a parent give up their child to a grave?

Parents ask why, but there is no answer to justify a child's death, no acceptable reason why a child should die. Parents ask, "Why me? Why did my child die? What is wrong with me? What did I do wrong?" They also contend with the questions that others ask them. Members of the extended family, neighbors, police, funeral directors, doctors, medical examiners ask, "Why? What happened? What did you do or neglect to do?" Blame will take over and begin to answer some of these questions, for no real explanation satisfies.

He whom we love and lose is no longer where he was before:
He is now wherever we are. *

The parents continue to care for their child despite his death, and they learn to find comfort in memories. Memories keep the dead alive, preserve and protect the lost loved one. Through memory the dead can be with us, wherever we are. Photographs and portraits along with clothing and small treasures are concrete memories. They are real and can be touched and held. Memories can be shared with others through stories and recollections of special days and events or words. The child can also be remembered in silence and solitude. The dead child is always part of one's memory and never forgotten.

In the process of mourning one's child, parents search for ways to fill some of their emptiness. They search for meaning, search for some justice in their injustice.

After a child has died, other children may be born into the family. The dead child cannot be replaced although a different child may be born or adopted. Joy will be felt for the new life and sadness will continue for the dead child. The wish for another child may be hampered by difficulty in conceiving or compounded by illness or discord in the parents' relationship. Some relationships may not be able to grow beyond the death of the child; separation or divorce may occur. The void between the parents deepens, leaving them far apart and unable to help each other or their relationship.

*Reprinted from the film, "When A Child Dies" with permission of the National Funeral Directors Association, Milwaukee.

Sometimes no meaning can be found in the child's death. This leaves little to hold on to for solace. If the child's life had been filled with pain and suffering from illness or the death was sudden or violent, parents will suffer in their knowledge of the anguish of the child's dying and death. If sweet and endearing memories can be recalled vividly, they offer support and serve to help with healing and living without.

The bereaved move on to the next day, week, month, year, decade, and after. While bereaved parents fill their lives in many areas, the empty space left by the child who has died is never filled. The empty space is forever. Happy and sad times will join in a peculiar kind of balance. The child's own days—birthday, the anniversary of his death, and other special moments—will be remembered vividly, with great sadness and longing, with signs of acute grief as though he just died, and with the joy of having him so much a part of one's self.

When a child dies, parents learn to live without him and live with him, knowing and feeling that their child is always with them, always a part of them.

And never forget, there is memory. . . .

—John Irving
The World According to Garp

From One Mom to Another
*by Netta Kandell**

Laura just left. It is 6:15 a.m., still dark outside. I thought I might go back to sleep, but no way . . . I am too excited.

. . . Laura has left before on other adventures, to camp, to her first day in school, even on an airplane once by herself when she was small. But, somehow it is different now. She is 13 years old and wants to do it all by herself. "Don't worry Mom, I'll be fine." How I remember saying that to you!!!

And, I really am *not* worried and am so proud that she wants to do it all herself. However, there is a leftover emotion that is difficult to define. I have an immediate instinct that you would understand that lingering feeling—well—how it is to be a Mom.

Laura will be gone for a week and, of course she will be back. But I know that she will be gone again and again, and each time she returns, it will probably be a little bit different.

Maybe it is the gray morning rapidly turning brighter, or the sleepy quiet of the early morning house . . . I am feeling, for the first time, the perspective of time, of how my child's life passes through mine, and of how she will someday be gone, "doing it all herself."

It is a good feeling. Laura is maturing and so healthy and eager. It is also an emotional knowledge that her time with me, as her Mom, as it has been so far, is really short, in the entire scheme of her life and mine.

Where is she going though? She is heading South to visit her grandparents, my parents, stepping back one generation for a time. That is right too, in the scheme of things, in her lifetime and yours.

I started this monologue thinking of me and what it is like to be a Mom. Now, I am thinking of you and your child, my brother, dead now 3 years. We don't talk about Alan as much as we think of him.

I know that he is gone, and the time he passed through your life was too short. As many times as he left "to do it himself" he always came back, and each time it was a little different. But Mom, that's how it is to be a Mom, even though his last departure was incomprehensible. Perhaps, from one Mom to another, I understand it all a little better now. The time we have with our children is limited; they must leave.

*Reprinted with permission from Netta Kandell.

The time we have with our children is forever, despite their leave. The time we have with our children is something to cherish.

I hope that I haven't caused you to feel sad. A child's leaving is part of a mother's possession. And to have that possession, no matter what may accompany it, is not sad, it is incredibly special.

I love you Mom.

Please give my child, also yours, a big hug and kiss for me. I do know that you cherish your time with her and also with me, your child. Perhaps that is why I *knew* you'd understand . . . so, that's how it feels to be a Mom.

Your daughter

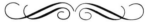

References

Irving, J. *The world according to Garp.* New York: E.P. Dutton, 1978.

Lindbergh, A.M. *Hour of gold, hour of lead: Diaries and letters of Anne Morrow Lindbergh. 1929-1932.* New York: Harcourt Brace Jovanovich, Inc., 1973.

Suggested Reading

Donnelly, K.F. *Recovering from the loss of a child.* New York: Macmillan, 1982.

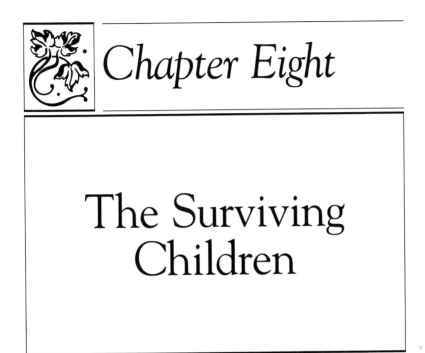

Chapter Eight

The Surviving Children

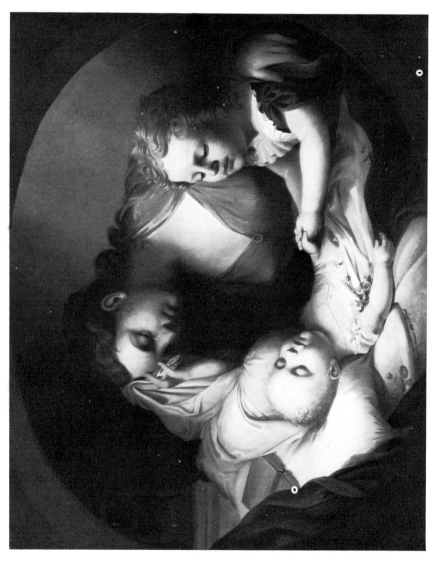

FREDERICK STILES AGATE, *Mother Lamenting over Her Dead Child*, 1827. Oil on Canvas. (Courtesy of the National Academy of

Agate's Mother lamenting over her child *depicts a young mother in sorrowful resignation and a despairing child mourning an infant in the sleep of death. The theme of the deceased child—popular in the nineteenth century—is underscored by an hourglass in the background, a symbol of the transcience of earthly life.* *

T HE DEARTH OF PROFESSIONAL LITERATURE HARDLY REFLECTS the significance of a sibling's death to the remaining child or children in a family. These survivors express in their behavior and in words the deeply felt impact.

There most certainly are short-term effects: horror, distress, and sadness. There is concern that what has happened to a brother or sister might in some way befall the surviving child. There is guilt that wishes, nasty thoughts, or words might have possessed a power strong enough to kill. There is the peculiar sense of relief in having mother and father home and physically in attendance as well as the disappointment at the parents' sadness and preoccupation with thoughts of the dead child. There are the personal feelings of loss of a special relationship; the pain of losing a loved brother or sister is profound.

The long-term effects are not as easy to identify and measure, for they last a lifetime. When questioned, adults remember vividly a sibling's death and often their own feelings with such clarity as if the

* From *all walks of life: Paintings of the figure from the National Academy of Design*, New York, 1979, p. 18.

death were yesterday. Personal experiences of many years ago are recalled in vivid and poignant detail, including feelings in response to the loss, the reactions of each parent to the death and to the remaining children. Emotions and powerful memories lie buried close to the surface and can be uncovered with surprising ease.

Because the death of a child member becomes part of the history of the family, a surviving child must in some way and at some time confront the sibling's death. This confrontation occurs whether or not the sibling's death has preceded the birth of the surviving child. Families struggle with this part of their history, commemorating the deceased child in words and pictures, remembering special days and events in his life, saving clothes and possessions, and counting him as one of the family members.

Communication patterns in a family determine the ease or difficulty with which the surviving members are able to live with the death and with their combined and separate mourning. If parents speak of the dead child, the sad and joyful memories, if they include his photographs in family clusters, they clearly give permission for the surviving siblings to remember, to ask questions, and to express the thoughts and wishes that linger. One family maintained a row of photographs arranged in chronological order in the family room. These were taken of the eight children at the time of birth. Adjacent to those were the most recent photographs. Striking in that lineup of cheery, healthy faces was the last photograph taken of the dead child. The siblings born after that death argued among themselves whether they would include him in the number eight or exclude him and not account for him. Loss in the family system has many interpretations; each sibling deals with the loss in relation to personal need and ways of coping and dealing with the reality.

The mother in this family maintained what she called a "cry box" containing all of the special possessions of the dead child from his kindergarten art productions to his infamous sneakers remembered by the family for their worndown, odoriferous state. The other children were invited to look at that box and tell or listen to stories about the contents and the child to whom they had belonged. Endless hours were spent with these pictures and possessions, and the dead child occupied a significant place within the family.

We Are Seven[*]

—A simple child,
That lightly draws its breath,
And feels its life in every limb,
What should it know of death?

I met a little cottage girl:
She was eight years old, she said;
Her hair was thick with many a curl
That clustered round her head.

She had a rustic, woodland air,
And she was wildly clad:
Her eyes were fair, and very fair;
—Her beauty made me glad.

"Sisters and brothers, little maid,
How many may you be?"
"How many? Seven in all," she said,
And wondering looked at me.

"And where are they? I pray you tell."
She answered, "Seven are we;
And two of us at Conway dwell,
And two are gone to sea.

"Two of us in the church-yard lie,
My sister and my brother;
And, in the church-yard cottage, I
Dwell near them with my mother."

"You say that two at Conway dwell,
And two are gone to sea,
Yet ye are seven! I pray you tell,
Sweet maid, how this may be."

Then did the little maid reply,
"Seven boys and girls are we;
Two of us in the church-yard lie,
Beneath the church-yard tree."

"You run about, my little maid,
Your limbs they are alive;
If two are in the church-yard laid,
Then ye are only five."

"Their graves are green, they may be seen,"
The little maid replied,
"Twelve steps or more from my mother's door,
And they are side by side.

"My stockings there I often knit,
My kerchief there I hem;
And there upon the ground I sit,
And sing a song to them.

"And often after sunset, Sir,
When it is light and fair,
I take my little porringer,
And eat my supper there.

"The first that died was sister Jane;
In bed she moaning lay,
Till God released her of her pain;
And then she went away.

"So in the church-yard she was laid;
And, when the grass was dry,
Together round her grave we played,
My brother John and I.

"And when the ground was white with snow,
And I could run and slide,
My brother John was forced to go,
And he lies by her side."

"How many are you, then," said I,
"If they two are in heaven?"
Quick was the little maid's reply,
"O Master we are seven."

"But they are dead; those two are dead!
Their spirits are in heaven!"
'Twas throwing words away; for still
The little maid would have her will,
And said, "Nay, we are seven!"

—William Wordsworth
(1770-1850)

[*]Reprinted from Houghton Mifflin Company, publishers, 1910. From *The Complete Poetical Works of William Wordsworth, Volume II, 1798-1800.*

Each child in a family has a special meaning and place. Families will recall that meaning with humor and sadness and with the myriad of intense emotions that continue for one who is dead. Usually in human interchange, there is a mutual and continuous interaction, allowing for change and growth; these times of reminiscing with the dead child's legacy prevent exchange and transformation, particularly if the dead child were never really known to the sibling.

The death of a child member of a family affects the parents' ability to respond to the remaining children and the quality of the response itself. Initially, at the time of death and for the acute period of mourning, parents may be quite unresponsive to remaining children, unavailable and detached, caught up in their own web of grief. The normal family exchanges around play, school, and everyday matters become unimportant.

The sharing of secrets, humorous happenings, and observations is avoided by parents whose energies are needed for recovery and healing or who may feel that to share joy would be unfair to their dead child. The presence of healthy children is both welcome and unwelcome. The healthy child is the bittersweet reminder of the lost health or vitality of the child who is dead.

Parents suffer a devastating and shattering blow to their own self-esteem, their sense of themselves as good parents. They feel that they have failed in their primary task to protect and sustain their children. The confusion and internal questioning that result affect the quality of their responses to their surviving children. These children feel parental ambivalence, the tentativeness of replies, the suspension of sure judgment. They experience distance and confusion. Some remaining children question their value to their parents, considering the devastation that they have witnessed in their parents' response to their sibling's death, and wonder why their love is not enough to fill their parents' emptiness.

There is a range of reactions to surviving children over time; these are dependent in part on the pattern and nature of the parents' grieving process, that is, how parents as individuals and as a couple deal with this loss. One father described his reluctance to spend time with his surviving son, seemingly frightened of the possibility of deepening this relationship and then losing this son.

Some parents describe themselves as being more cautious than ever protecting their remaining children. Activities and experiences formerly encouraged are forbidden for fear of injury. Children are kept from areas where contamination or hurt might occur; threats may be exaggerated and distorted by the parent as they make day-to-day judgments about the safety of their surviving children.

Following the death of children, parents may consider conceiving another child immediately or adopting a child to fill the empty place that exists in the family. One father commented that should his seriously ill son die, he would adopt a boy of the same age and coloring. Indeed he would name him for his dead child and expect of him similar attributes. Other families listening to this father responded in horror but then acknowledged their understanding of his wish to provide an exact substitute for his dying son.

In a more subtle substitution process, some parents will endow their surviving children with the qualities and attributes of the dead child and will have the same expectations of the living children as they had of the one now dead. That this child cannot live up to those expectations or may exceed them is a constant source of disappointment to parents, whose need is to protect themselves from the pain of their grief.

Many families find in their remaining children comfort and solace and reason to go on. In an effort to confirm their capabilities as parents to their remaining children, there may be perceptible changes in their availability and care. One father left his position as an executive officer in a company and preferred to work in a less demanding position, desiring more time and energy for his family after his young son died. This father stated that his own perception of his living child changed and he treasured the time spent with her.

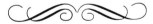

SIBLINGS' RESPONSES

Thoughts of a Sister*
by Lorraine Anne Szybist

I have tried to talk about my brother's death with other people. My grandmother gets upset and sounds as if she's going to cry, even now. What she remembers is his smile, and then she wonders why God took him away. My dad doesn't talk about it at all. I've tried to ask him questions, but I can tell he doesn't want to think about it. My dad was with me and my brother when my brother died, and I think that still bothers him. My mom is the only one I can talk to about my brother. She listens and tells me how she feels, too. I'm glad that someone will talk to me about it and feel that what I have to say is important. I think that's good, because I also need someone to talk to sometimes. When we talk about how I reacted, it seems as if we are talking about another person entirely. It's strange to imagine that it really all happened. My mom told me that she didn't take me to the funeral. I don't remember that, but it makes me mad now to think that they left me home with someone else. It sometimes amazes me how freely my mom can talk to me about my brother when I ask. I'm glad that she can. But I've also noticed something else. Every year around the time of my brother's birthday, my mom gets weird. I don't know how else to explain it, but I know she must think about him alot then. And it was so long ago! She doesn't cry. It's just something that I feel must be happening to her. That bothers me alot.

I have a brother who was born after Larry died. He's 8 years old, and if someone mentions Larry to him, he gets upset. That puzzles me because he wasn't even alive when Larry died. I wonder if he acts upset because he really is or if he feels he should be upset. When we get mad at each other and fight, sometimes I tell him that I wish that he had died instead of Larry. That makes him even madder. Sometimes he tells me that he wishes I were dead. Neither one of us means it, and maybe if we hadn't lost a brother, we would say those kinds of things to each other and they wouldn't mean anything. I don't know. . . .

Maybe if my brother hadn't died, I wouldn't be afraid to babysit. And maybe if my brother hadn't died, we wouldn't have the brother I

*At the time of writing, the author was a high-school student. Reprinted with permission from Sahler, Olle Jane Z., editor: *The child and death,* St. Louis, 1978, The C.V. Mosby Co. and with permission from the author and editor.

have now, and I wouldn't like that. I think that maybe there were some good things, though. We all care about each other a lot. Maybe we would have done that anyway. Mostly when I think about my brother, what I really feel is that something is missing.

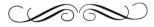

There is little discussion in the literature of the impression and impact of funeral and burial attendance on the surviving children. There is a paucity of material to guide parents with the very difficult decisions that they must make for their other children when one child dies. (See Appendix for suggested readings.) At best, there is controversy about the value of siblings participating in funeral and burial rituals. Few guidelines are offered to assist families in the decision making. Usually discussion involves analysis of the issue in relation to developmental abilities of particular growth and development periods of childhood. Key to all analyses of this issue is the importance of the support that these children need from their parents throughout the funeral rituals. An indication of the family's ability to sustain and support is seen in the child's willingness to attend the funeral. The child's wishes must be listened to carefully.

Some participation in the family's rituals of mourning serves to include the remaining children in a process that allows them and the parents to begin to live without the dead child and to strengthen their relationships as survivors who must continue to live productively together. To be excluded from the critical events following the death widens the gap between grieving parents and surviving children. These early decisions and the degree of sharing the grief set the stage for how the loss will be dealt with in the weeks, months, and years ahead. Exclusion itself is a statement of parental detachment and isolation. The children left out can think only of their presence as being unimportant, providing no comfort. They are demeaned; their own sadness and distress go unrecognized.

Some parents may arrange with their clergy or a significant support person to meet with them and their children before the traditional funeral service for prayer, quiet discussion, and a time of shared sadness. The family shares this special time together, allowing the children to question, cry, perhaps to touch the coffin or flowers and see the body if they wish.

Careful description and explanation geared to the child's understanding of what he will see and hear as well as the opportunity to review his impressions and perceptions afterward are important for children of all ages. This principle also applies to the explanation of the cause and circumstances of the death. If parents are entangled in their own grief so that they are unable to provide this closeness and comfort, a family friend or relative who knew both the dead child and the living, as well as the family's religious or ideological beliefs and feelings, may be in a position to assist the surviving children or help by encouraging the parents to share their grief. In this way, strength is gained from the love among the family members.

Surviving children sorely miss their dead sibling. Longing for his presence and companionship will continue over a lifetime. The remaining children struggle with issues of responsibility and guilt for their imagined or actual participation in the death of their sibling. The normal and universal feelings of rivalry become painfully accentuated when a sister or brother is sick over some time, requiring parental attention and concern. What of the angry thoughts and wishes provoked by the sick child in a moment of teasing or rage? What of the hostile acts that may in fact have contributed to a sibling's death?

There may be an enormous burden of guilt to be carried by the child whose action or whose inability to protect contributed to a sibling's death. For children whose guilt is great by virtue of their own fantasies or real actions, the need for careful discussing and listening is pressing.

This work, which may include the parents, often must be done with the aid of a therapist, who can respond from a more neutral base than family members. Whatever the circumstances, the guilt will not dissipate. These feelings need to be worked through carefully and sensitively.

Surviving siblings may respond by emulating the behaviors and mannerisms of the dead child. As an immediate response, it is protective and may elicit the praise and comfort of understanding adults and win a special place for the child in the family. Over the long period of time, it may be burdensome, impede growth, and influence the development of the surviving child.

Children whose siblings die of difficult and painful diseases often develop a hypochondriacal response, imitating the physical neediness of the ill child and unconsciously substituting their own concerns for those of the parent who is emotionally distant and preoccupied. These children may express untoward fear of bodily injury or illness as a statement of their own heightened vulnerability.

Remaining children may confound and anger parents in their ability to maintain academic performance, to enjoy peers and activities, to contribute to the family, and to continue to grow despite having lost a sibling. Indeed some children demonstrate a perceptible amount of growth in maturity. A family may denounce these responses as being egocentric, proving that the remaining sibling is unfeeling, insincere, or callous.

Some appreciation of the fact that children mourn but mourn differently than adults is important. A child can continue about the business of play and work without the incumbrance of constant, unrelenting grief. For the surviving child or children the grieving process seems to be dealt with little by little rather than as the more continuous process for the adult. In children reworking can occur sporadically and spontaneously when memories of the dead brother or sister are touched. The nature of childhood bereavement is reflected in a combination of factors including the developmental level, what the family will allow, and the child's own special style of relating and dealing with the world. Each family member—adult and child—grieves differently for the lost member. They grieve for the dead child, for themselves, and for the changed family system.

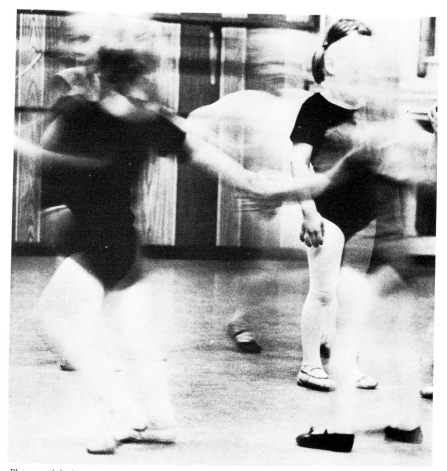

Photograph by Karen Dusenbery. (Courtesy of St. Louis Information and Counseling Program for Sudden Infant Death.)

Suggested Readings

Cain, A.C., Fast, I., and Erickson, M. Children's disturbed reactions to the death of a sibling. *American Journal of Orthopsychiatry,* 1964, *34,* 741-752.

Feinberg, D. Preventive therapy with siblings of a dying child. *Journal of the American Academy of Child Psychiatry,* 1970, 9(4), 644-668.

Krell, R., and Rabkin, L. The effects of sibling death on the surviving child: A family perspective. *Family Process,* December 1979, *18,* 471-477.

Moriarity, I. Mourning the death of an infant: The siblings' story. *The Journal of Pastoral Care,* March 1978, *32,* 22-33.

Plank, E., and Prank, R. Children and death. *The Psychoanalytic Study of the Child,* 1978, *33,* 593-620.

Sahler, O.J.Z. (Ed.). *The child and death.* St. Louis: C.V. Mosby Co., 1978.

Schowalter, J.E. Children and funerals. *Pediatrics in Review,* April 1980, *1,* 337-339.

Schowalter, J.E. How do children and funerals mix? *Journal of Pediatrics,* 1976, *89,* 139-142.

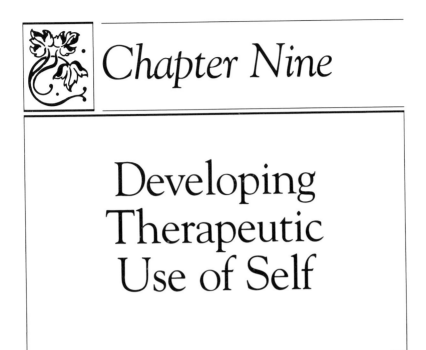

Chapter Nine

Developing Therapeutic Use of Self

W E IN THE HELPING FIELDS HAVE COME TO UNDERSTAND
something about the significance of the loss of a loved one and the
process of mourning such a loss. Touching on the fringes of the
intensity of grief, we are trying to make sense of it, to deepen our
understanding so that we can be as helpful as possible in our approach
as caregivers. But we are all beginners in this process. There are no
absolute answers or protocols on which to rely. There are no remedies
or cures. Rather, we learn through involvement with grieving families. Our learning is continuous and new. The more we know from
families, the more we are awed by the intensity of grief and humbled
by the lessons of the bereaved.

The death of a child is the most severe crisis and the most
significant loss for a family. This is true regardless of the age of the
child, the circumstances of the death—whether sudden or
expected—or the cause of the death. When a child dies is not
predictive of the intensity of the grief response. It is no more or less
painful if a child dies at 3 months, 3 years, 30 years, or 60 years of age.
It is the very fact that a *child* has died that is profound and different
from other deaths. The cause and the circumstances of each child's
death are unique.

If days and months or even years pass as a child is dying, the family may have the opportunity to share and anticipate the death. When the child dies, however, grieving does not end. Parents continue to grieve throughout their lives. No reason justifies the death of a child. Whether death is caused by an accident, a chronic disease, a sudden and rapid illness, suicide, or an unexplained syndrome or situation, child death is unjustified and incomprehensible, an unnecessary ending of a young life. Each family is left to deal with the circumstances and the cause of the death as only they can, as best they can. The whys will never be answered.

The dead child is mourned forever. Parents cannot accept their child's death. A parent may in some way learn to live without the child and to live with the emptiness—what the child was and could have been. But these families are never whole again; nothing said or done can restore them to wholeness. We can help. We can assist families in sorting out, understanding, and expressing feelings, and we can support the members as they learn to live without their dead child and with each other in a productive and meaningful way.

To do this, we need to begin within ourselves; we need to examine our thoughts and feelings about a child's death and the bereaved family. Often a family grieving their dead child is judged, and the quality of parenting is questioned. Parents assume responsibility for their children, so their sense of responsibility is challenged. We ask if they acted appropriately and soon enough. We ask, "Why them? What makes them different?" We wonder what went wrong, what they did or did not do that was wrong. These questions and doubts are communicated overtly and covertly.

As caregivers we need to start within ourselves by examining our preconceived ideas and judgments. This influence may be subtle or pervasive, but the influence will be felt. This self-examination is particularly important because the very essence of our interactions with families is the therapeutic use of ourselves. We as caregivers can never know enough about mourning. The more we comprehend, the more we realize that we can never completely know and understand the pain and reactions of another. People touch us and we touch them in the process of sharing the pain of their loss. Yet as much as we share, we really do not know their pain.

We do gain strength from each other, from within ourselves, and by sharing. We know only the periphery or the surface of the meaning of another's loss. Further, there are no words to describe the pain of losing a child. Part of it cannot ever be shared.

Anger is part of the grieving response and yet it often takes us by surprise. It can frighten and distance the helper—especially if the anger is taken personally, signifying rejection. The family may be blaming the health care system for its neglect, for not keeping their child alive. Anger is an expression of powerlessness and helplessness. Dealing with anger becomes a vehicle in assisting the family to cope with their grieving more effectively. Expressing anger may be a way of asking for help. As caregivers we can offer ourselves, our skilled ears to listen carefully, and our sensitivity and concern as we reach out to be with the bereaved. We are there to listen, to look with families at their strengths and alternatives, to promote an atmosphere of acceptance and appreciation of the meaning of their loss, and to provide an environment to facilitate the expression of grief among family members. As caregivers our concern is the health of people—individuals, families, groups, and communities. We seek knowledge to help us learn more about our clients' needs, how to help them when their health is threatened, and how to provide appropriate and meaningful care.

When do we take the time to discuss our needs, our feelings, our reactions to situations, to understand our strengths and our limitations? Working with families in grief is very special. We get close to people during the worst tragedy in their lives. We treat wounds that never completely heal, wounds that result in excruciating pain. Working with families in grief means expressing our humanity, trying to empathize. As we share ourselves we also share in their tragedy. We enter another's space dominated by grief. We come close to facing death. We are also reminded of the quality of life. We become impressed with the quickness of our lives. We hear the clock tick, recognize the need to value each day, and try to keep close to the people whom we love—ever mindful of the care and effort needed to maintain these relationships. We are also impressed with the mundane, with the ease of getting caught in a web of complexities and trivia, and with the passage of days turned into years. We are reminded of our losses, the death of people whom we have loved deeply. We are reminded as well of the unresolved relationships, the words never spoken, the inner peace that might have been, the sadness and longing for, the emptiness. We think of the conflict, anger, and resentment never dealt with adequately.

Perhaps we too have suffered the death of a child, a child for whom we grieve all the days of our lives; the pain of that loss collides with the feelings that others may share with us. Along with our concern we bring our personal histories of loss and longing for those whom we love who have died. We bring our pain, and we are reminded of our own vulnerability that death can come to us and to someone whom we love dearly in the unpredictable future. We dread the loss of connectedness that death causes and recognize that mourning is an attempt to keep connected, to keep alive our loving and caring, and to continue our relationships in some way with those whom we have lost to death. We face our own fears and fantasies and know that the sadness within us will be grabbed at and pulled to the surface when we work with and know of people in grief.

In working with the bereaved we come with our

- hurts and losses,
- feelings about loss by death,
- desire to care for others,
- ability to reach out and involve ourselves, and
- inability when overpowered by the horror of a child's death and our own sadness.

One of the authors recalls a situation from her own personal experience as the coordinator of a counseling program on infant death:

> Our office was located in the morgue—and we were to provide on-site counseling for families who came to identify their dead infants. One of our responsibilities was to accompany the family to view their dead child. In spite of the many families who had described their baby's death to me, I had not seen their

dead child. This escorting of families was one of my almost daily functions. Each time I took a parent to the viewing room, I felt uncomfortable. I wanted the viewing to be as brief as possible. I focused on the difficulties that *I* felt parents must be having with the experience. Once while alone with a baby, rearranging the blanket that covered his body, I realized what was troubling me. I was afraid of his dead body, afraid to touch death—to come too close to death. From that point, my conflict about the viewing was relieved; I was more comfortable within myself and consequently I was able to be with families more concerned with their experience, and less concerned with protecting myself. I was able to stay with families and listen to them speak about or to their dead child or simply stand in silence as they stared at or touched him.

This account conveys the necessity of recognizing personal fears and reactions as well as limitations while working with bereaved families. Our feelings and fears will surface whether or not we choose to deal with them. As they surface, our reactions and abilities will be altered.

In fact, caregivers in the process of self-exploration need to analyze their motives for working with bereaved families. Issues from our past can guide or provide direction for each of us in the professional decisions that we make. Much remains unexplained or appears unconnected as we work and apply our energies in the service of others who are bereaved. Regardless, this analysis of our own life of losses is essential and basic to the process of caring. In this we are truly caring for ourselves and building an ability to care for another. This analysis promotes objectivity, which is important in a therapeutic relationship. We are therefore responsible and accountable for exploring our beliefs about death, loss, bereavement; about children, families, parenting; about children dying; and about our need to help, to be helpful to others.

As caring professionals we want to help; we want to heal hurts and eliminate pain; we want to correct, to restore, to make whole again, to alter somehow the course of events that led to this end. In child death, we cannot accomplish these tasks, and it helps to accept this reality. We can act through understanding, believing in the strengths of people to survive and live on, to rebuild their sense of self-esteem as parents and lovers, restoring meaning and significance in their relationships as well as creating new ones.

Recommending solutions often comes too easily to helpers. We offer answers to the situation as we perceive it, solutions that make sense to us. Rather, we need to look through the eyes and feel through the senses of the family, to listen and believe in their ability to choose and act for themselves. This approach in itself is therapeutic. Empathy is not possible in this instance, but we can try to work toward it. In no way can we feel the intensity of the loss or know what it is like to live through time after the death of one's child. In truth, the caregiver cannot experience the pain nor take the pain away. The caregiver may help the client to speak of the pain, to understand it, and to live with it. For the caregiver there is this tug-of-war in bereavement work. There is the desire to extend oneself and share in the pain of another and to pull back because the pain is so big and consuming and frightening. Child death affects us all.

The therapeutic process begins by acknowledging that the death of a child is undoubtedly the ultimate tragedy; children are not supposed to die. The process of helping is an interactional process, the interactions and interrelationships of people reaching out to each other. For the caregiver, this assumes the need for openness and a willingness to become involved. No one emerges ready to do this work. We all must start somewhere; it is always difficult to begin. There is little balance in this work; it involves being exposed to a great deal of hurt, powerlessness, rage, and emptiness. It means voluntarily putting ourselves in a hurting place. We must attempt to feel what it is like to lose a child, whether we have children or not. In addition, our clients let us know about their needs and pain, but they may not always let us know when they are all right or better. When a family calls 6 months or 1 year or 10 years after a child's death, one expects that it is a call for help. It may be a difficult anniversary, a particularly agonizing time of emptiness and longing.

Being able to extend oneself in this interactional process of helping requires the ability to share and yet to remain separate. That separateness allows the caregiver to give care to another in a selfless way so that the client's needs are primary. It is separateness that allows the caregiver to be a careful listener.

To work in this capacity over time, we must take into account our needs. It helps to provide a regular time to listen to each other and to share feelings, to aid in each other's refueling. We must take the initiative to care for ourselves so that we can feel good about ourselves and our work. It is the unique agency or institution that has a support network for care providers built into the practice setting. It is also important to build collaborative relationships with colleagues so that they are available to relieve us or spell us when we feel overwhelmed. We need to allow ourselves to request help. A person cannot keep fresh and sensitive each moment. We need solitude and time in the form of holidays and vacations to rekindle our energies and deal with our feelings. Most of all, we need balance and perspective to help us know that children are born to grow and flourish and not to die.

No one is unaffected by loss or exempt from feelings of grief. Sharing feelings, building collaborative networks, taking time away are essential life supports for the caregiver of the bereaved. Without these supports, distancing oneself, becoming detached, disengaged, impersonal, even unavailable are ways of trying to protect oneself from hurt. We do not choose whether or not we should grieve; we do grieve. Without taking care of ourselves or without breaks or balance in our work we may begin to experience a sense of being dissipated. We may begin to see ourselves as failures, develop negative feelings about ourselves, experience conflict in both personal and professional relationships. We may begin to feel a dehumanizing effect, losing sight of the client as a real person and seeking to distance ourselves from the client, not really making contact. We may feel great anger at our clients and guilt for harboring such resentment.

These feelings find expression in family and professional relationships. Some of the warning signs of feeling depleted include experiencing chronic exhaustion, feeling upset, having difficulty eating or sleeping or experiencing frequent nightmares, developing psychosomatic symptoms (headaches, backaches, weakness), feeling physically and emotionally exhausted, unhappy, trapped, worthless, rejected, pessimistic. The emotionally depleted caregiver may begin to avoid contact with others, leave work early, and arrive late.

There is also the potential for the caregiver to lose a personal sense of self and move in with the family. The boundaries that serve to separate effectively one person from another to maintain individual identity begin to loosen. The caregiver can get lost and not be able to navigate through the morass of sadness, thereby relinquishing the ability to guide and anticipate in this relationship, which has lost its therapeutic quality. Further, we may encourage families to become reliant or dependent on us. Dependency in relationships without limits of time and space is not therapeutic.

The caregiver therefore must enter a helping relationship with a healthy sense of respect for the client as a separate person capable of independent decisions and self-care. The fulfillment of a therapeutic relationship lies in the following:

- To try to be empathic or move toward empathy in order to comprehend the magnitude of the loss to the family on the death of their child.

- To be accepting and unafraid, not rejecting and limiting.

- To listen and to speak of child death, recognizing it for all that it is—an unparalleled human tragedy. To ensure that families will be respected and admired for their ability to deal with the vastness of their loss, we need to legitimize their loss, to talk openly about the dead child. To continue the silence is somehow to deny the child's very existence and to deny the parents their relationship with this special person who lived, was a significant part of their lives, and has a place within them as long as they live.

- To attempt to resolve our own fears about death, our sense of intruding into an area of people's lives that we construe as private, intimate, and personal. Grief can be shared. We need to be hopeful, still recognizing their feelings of hopelessness, knowing that families can survive.

- To believe in the families' strengths and abilities to cope, to take charge of their shattered lives again, to make decisions, and to rebuild self-esteem as effective parents.

- To foster and maximize these strengths and existing networks of support. We need to encourage families to rely on their own good judgment and make the most of the supportive ties and connections that they already possess but may not be utilizing fully, and to seek new avenues of support.
- To serve as a facilitator for effective communication among family members by listening, clarifying, promoting, and encouraging interchange.

Through this we support families as they learn to live with their pain and live without their child.

As families search for meaning, so do caregivers. We can find meaning through the sharing of our humanity, by building connections between people, and by facing openly our own feelings about child death. The foundations for working with grieving families are the caring and open attitude with which we come and the desire to listen, understand, appreciate, and accept feelings and experiences. No one person is better prepared to deal with grieving families than another. Grief and loss are not the focus of any one discipline. In truth, each of us has something unique to offer. We offer ourselves. There are no answers and no explanations adequate to justify the injustice of losing a child. But involvement, the sharing of one's humanity, will make a difference.

Suggested Reading

Havens, L. The existential use of self. *The American Journal of Psychiatry*, January 1974, *131*(1), 1-10.

Chapter Ten

Working with Bereaved Families

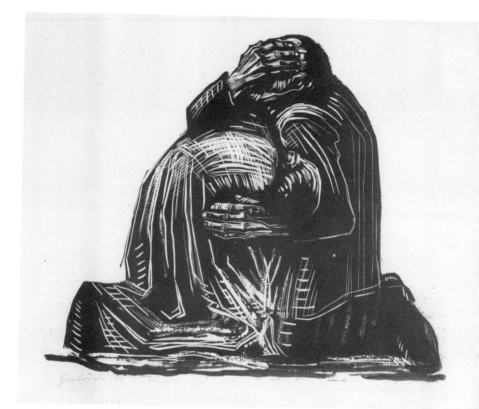

KATHE KOLLWITZ, *The Parents.* Woodcut, 1923. (Photograph courtesy Galerie St. Etienne, New York)

APPROACHING THE FAMILY

Beginning to work with a family involves internaliz-
ing a belief that a child's death has a profound impact on the family
and that recognition, acceptance, and validation of their experience
are means of providing needed support for the anguished family.
Beginning means wanting to be with and available to the family in
grief. Their pain may be overpowering, even consuming, yet the
caregiver approaches them. Fear and helplessness may emerge within
the caregiver from a feeling of impotency in facing the power of
another's grief. The caregiver enters a space of pain filled with
sadness, emptiness, desperation, confusion, and rage.

It is often difficult to begin; who would willingly subject himself to
this pain? It is no wonder that those in grief are so often asked to
forget their lost loved one and go on with life. The bereaved are asked
to put away their pain because it is intolerable to the onlooker, who
may feel drained, emptied, reminded of his own losses, and threatened by his vulnerability. In this close relationship with death, the
caregiver may also be reminded of the precious nature of life itself,
feel its wonder, and value his own loved ones.

Being available to another in grief means lending oneself to another. Nothing can be asked of the bereaved family. Having no expectations, the caregiver has no preconceived thoughts or images of how one should look or behave when a child dies. Grief is not uniform; rather, it is a statement of an individual's coping, and there is a wide range of normal coping behaviors.

As a helper, the caregiver is oriented toward caring and curing, making better or easier, and alleviating another's suffering. Yet in grief work, the caregiver can make no promise of alleviation or relief of pain. Rather, the focus of the interaction is to assist family members in living with this pain, living with their loss. The caregiver serves as a facilitator for the expressions of their grief. Working with bereaved families means accepting that the family is free to share what they choose while the caregiver's responsibility is to work with what is given. The surfaced part of the experience can be shared; the depths of grief cannot be shared.

If we begin with our concern for the family, then the family will provide the direction for our interactions. Families teach about their needs and guide the caregiver in offering support appropriately. The family can be asked what kind of help is needed. Often these needs may be very different than the proposed solutions that another may offer.

Families are able to make decisions in their own time and own way. Nevertheless, it is essential for the caregiver to reach out. Bereaved family members are not likely to call for assistance or for validation of their experience. Often their feelings of pain are so intense that the line between sanity and madness becomes indistinguishable. They may feel that they are losing their minds. It simply may require more energy than possible for the depleted parent to reach out for support. Decision making is especially difficult when dealing with loss. Reaching out to families is necessary. Home visits are particularly useful because care is brought to the doorstep, and the family maintains control since the caregiver is a guest. The family may not choose to return to the hospital where their child died, even if support is needed, because this journey is too painful. Outreach is required also because a common response in dealing with the death of one's child is to move; the members are unable to remain in their home confronted with so many reminders of the dead child. Often families stay with relatives or friends or even drift aimlessly, unable to return home.

Listening

No one is really expert in the field of bereavement; little research has been conducted to identify proven strategies for work with bereaved families. We are all learning. Listening to the best teachers, the families themselves, will enable the caregiver to learn in some small way about the enormous nature of grief when a child dies. Interacting means engaging in a mutual relationship, becoming involved, and giving and receiving. We convey our concern by giving of ourselves and accepting their pain. Through the process of talking about the death of one's child, feelings are recognized and legitimized; support is gained. The caregiver can feel restored by experiencing the strength of others in surviving.

The caregiver accepts the family and their responses without question. Families are diverse in their individual styles, methods of operating, values, rules, patterns. So too are grief responses unique. The caregiver accepts any possible grief reaction—anger, frustration, defeat, depression. The family may openly welcome the caregiver to share in their grief or close off attempts at establishing a relationship. Often parents are filled with guilt and spend years in anguish because they feel that if they had been better to their child, better parents, loved him more or protected him more, he would be alive. Listening involves using an astute ear for blame. Blame is always inner-directed and/or may be displaced on others. The parent without funds or appropriate insurance sought medical care, but the care may have been substandard; he blames the provider and also blames himself for not having the resources to secure the best health care for the child.

Accepting the Family Feelings

Caregivers frequently become scapegoats for parental rage even if they never knew or cared for the child, simply because they represent the health care system that could not prevent the child from dying and therefore become a source for parental anguish. It is difficult not to reject and to be open and accepting when rage is personally directed. It helps to recognize that horrifying powerlessness, loss of control, and painful yearning that lie beneath this surface expression. Behind the outbursts of anger are tears of helplessness that have not been given the opportunity to emerge. Anger may be the only sense of strength that the grieving parent feels he possesses.

The caregiver can assist the family members through acceptance and recognition of the intensity of their feelings and significance of their loss and by assisting them to identify and clarify their many strengths. Offering solutions to identified problems does not necessarily assist the family to mobilize those needed strengths to survive and grow together. As the caregiver listens, he can help the family members listen to themselves and identify alternatives for themselves. This approach also encourages communication within the family, fosters understanding through sharing, and reduces blame. Helping is a process not measured by the success or failure of outcomes.

Listening is an expression of concern. The caregiver communicates that he is with the family by leaning forward, establishing eye contact, reacting to the pain expressed, perhaps touching, and conveying through acceptance a trusting attitude. Listening means hearing what is said—the themes of guilt and blame, the problems. The family may be stricken with problems different from the child's death and yet paramount. If not attended to and remedied, grieving for the dead child may be forestalled or hampered.

The caregiver supports the parents by communicating a belief in their ability to parent effectively by admiring their strengths and love in caring for the other children and through recognition of their love for the dead child. Communicating with the bereaved family involves

- accepting,
- believing,
- clarifying,

- validating, and
- trusting.

The caregiver seeks to work with the whole family so that members talk and listen to each other, clarify each others' views and beliefs, understand their differences and learn to communicate the variety of feelings they experience. The caregiver senses from the family their desire to continue the process within the relationship, their readiness to explore feelings, and cope with their pain.

It is difficult to touch people in grief. The bereaved are lost in the depths of themselves and cannot always be summoned. When a child dies, the parent is lost, searching within for a reason, hoping to find some way to make the nightmare end. It is also difficult work because we do not want to touch such sadness and pain and because the agony affects us and makes us ache and recoil to protect ourselves and our loved ones.

FOCUSING WITH THE FAMILY

The grieving process is complex. The numerous variables in this process include family interaction, social interaction and support, previous grief patterns, cultural norms, and view of the future. The process of grieving does not progress in predictable sequential order. Grieving is not an all-or-nothing phenomenon. Some expressions of grief can be observed interacting simultaneously or a person can exhibit difficulty in moving beyond denial of the death. Responses are varied. The grief process in its complexities collides with the complexities and uniqueness of the individual in grief and in particular with the pieces of the past that each member carries. The parent brings his childhood. As adults we work on the child within us all the time and can well remember the powerlessness of being a child. As parents we are responsible for caring for that helpless and struggling child. The child is part of the parents' consciousness and the parent is within the child.

The focuses of the family in response to the loss of a child member are multiple, change with time, and vary in intensity. Each member of the family is affected by the death, and each will deal with the loss differently. These differences are often the cause of distance and misunderstanding. The caregiver can help each member appreciate that the other is grieving and recognize the way that each expresses himself. We idealize harmonious relationships but because of our normal differences, dysynchronous patterns are usually more common. The communication gap widens and needs are more exaggerated; disappointment and feelings of rejection become stronger. In working with the bereaved, it is important to recognize feelings and the differences in their expression. This approach will assist family members in deepening the bonds between them rather than widening the gaps.

Often feelings are put away to try to quiet the storm within only to find that it rages again in some crisis situation, like a subsequent pregnancy. This is especially true when the reality hits that soon a child will be born and the possibility of this child dying too comes closer and closer. It is not uncommon for siblings to feel directly responsible for the death of their brother or sister. Each member of the family wonders why. Grandparents grieve the loss of their grandchild as well as witness the death of part of their own child and also grieve this loss. Grandparents may wish that they could give their own life in exchange for the child. They bargain, feeling that they have lived long enough. If the grandparents were the primary caretaker of the child, this adds yet another dimension to their loss.

Families are systems. Families have their own patterns, boundaries, and power. The family is more than and different from the sum total of the individuals who comprise it. We cannot lump individual expressions into a family expression of grief. Similarly we cannot assume that fathers and mothers feel the same after their child's death. Nor can we exclude brothers and sisters, regardless of their ages, from personal grief. The family may also include extended family members, friends, and others who become natural support networks. All grieve for the dead child.

The family system changes when a child member dies. When a member of this system dies, the survivors must reorder the system, restructure it so that it continues to work for them. In a sense then, the energy for restructuring is part of the work of grieving, that is, it is energy needed to reorder one's life and integrate this loss into living and functioning. Since death remains a crisis in the system, inherent in this introduced change are the possibilities for creative alternatives in response to the change. If the family is using its energies to deal with the change and the intensity of meaning that it has for them as individuals and family members, this energy can be repatterned or rechanneled to promote a healthy family system. The caregiver may serve as a catalyst for communication and direction within the system.

A child's death affects the whole family. Often one can observe a balancing of roles within the family. For example, the father may listen and support the mother in her need to talk about their child and her fears and guilt while she supports him by dealing with the many telephone calls from family and friends. In healthy relationships roles tend to be reciprocal. When their child dies, it is helpful if the scales can be tilted and balanced to allow each partner the necessary release. It is helpful to act between them, easing the pressure and providing them with a new view of each other. Their communications will increase and they will be better able to respect and appreciate their differences and provide each other with needed space. Often this can be catalyzed by the presence of an objective person, while it would be impossible if they were alone because of their reliance on the pattern in their relationship. Equally important is preventing the caregiver from becoming part of a triangle with the couple. The caregiver becomes involved with the family primarily to encourage them to relate more meaningfully with each other, not to relate through another person.

Children in the household will be strongly affected by the death. The surviving child may feel guilt because he feels responsible for the death. One seven-year-old was able to say that she felt that it was her fault that the baby died. The evening her baby sister died she had stayed overnight at a friend's apartment. This was her first time sleeping at a friend's home. Usually she shared a bedroom with her baby sister. Her conviction was that she could have saved her sibling had she been home.

Parents very often need a great deal of help in planning how to handle the other children's reactions and interpretations of death. It is helpful to use the word *dead*, to understand that although young children do not comprehend death as permanent, they frequently feel that they too will die. Above all they need to feel safe, secure, and loved. Children often cling to their parents, thinking that if they are nearby, nothing will happen to them. Parents may find this very comforting but also very difficult when depleted; questions seem endless and the parents are tearful at the mention of the dead child's name. If the other children feel loved and safe, then they become more secure in the fact that they will not just disappear like their brother or sister did.

If parents want another child soon, they may find it helpful to know that this child is different. They will feel joy for the new life and sadness because they will continue to feel the pangs of loss for their dead child. In addition, they will be fearful that this child will also die.

Another reaction may involve sexual concerns. Touching and pleasing each other may be difficult for parents when reminded that their child is dead. If the mother or father feels that another child is out of the question, sexual abstinence may result in order to eliminate the possibility of another pregnancy. It is not uncommon for couples to feel differently about a subsequent child. One partner may want another baby and the other may feel the only way that they can cope is to prevent this. The caregiver can assist the couple to recognize their differences and the reasons underlying these differences. Discussion of anatomy, physiology, and birth control can be helpful. Sexual expression is a form of communication that is an important part of a relationship.

Often the emergent theme for the role of caregiver is the reinforcement of the individual's and family's strength and alternatives. Frequently, grieving parents are blind to the strengths and assets that they truly do possess. It is crucial not to minimize a parent's situation in any way, especially with phrases like "you are young" or "you can have another child." Avoiding euphemisms is necessary. Parents often feel that they have failed so profoundly as parents that their actions or omissions took their child's life. Identifying strengths helps in the healing process.

Individual and family coping behavior vary also with cultural beliefs and mores about what is acceptable and appropriate and how the period of grieving is managed. Grief for a child ignores all boundaries; reactions and responses will differ from person to person, family to family, culture to culture. One cannot measure the degree of pain or the significance of the lost child by expressed behavior alone. Expressions of grief may be dictated by family rules and societal values of acceptable behavior and may be very different from the caregiver's beliefs and practices. Shock and disbelief are necessary and serve to protect the family from the reality of loss. This numbing effect will alter natural responses. What is felt in grief is indescribable anyway.

The family in grief will contend with many experiences with the world outside, with others' perceptions and reactions. They may be feared or avoided. They may be blamed or expected to forget and put away their sorrow. They may be asked to fill themselves up again either with another child, a hobby, a new responsibility, a job, because their pain is communicated and the recipient may already feel drained and unable to be available for them. They may be held responsible for their child's death, for failing as parents; they may be accused of doing something wrong or of not caring enough. There may be no reason or rationale for this blame, but the parents are held responsible as others are threatened by the child's death.

True support is difficult to give because it means listening, accepting, and encouraging the family. Support comes without question or questioning unless these prove helpful to the family. Connections with available networks of support can be helpful. The parents require ties with life. Otherwise they have no reason to live. Families without available natural supports need to be connected to caring people and agencies by referral (Donnelly, 1982). Follow-up must also be ensured, otherwise the bereaved are at risk.

WORKING WITH THE FAMILY OVER TIME

While the caregiver may not in truth be able to join with the bereaved parent in the experience of losing his child, he can be with the parent in the realization of their powerlessness. That seems to be the place where all can join hands and minds and feelings.

Encounters with the bereaved family may be short or long, immediate or years after the child's death. Regardless, the operating principles are relatively constant. The caregiver engages in the human experience of reaching out to another and communicating in a helpful and healing way by exploring issues, opening communication, and offering information that may assist the family in anticipating and dealing with their grief reactions and experience. The caregiver promotes an atmosphere for expressing grief. Regardless of when the caregiver begins to work with the family in grief, they have felt, thought, and heard a variety of reactions and responses to their child's death and come to their own unique conclusions. Each family has a story to tell, a tragically painful story of all that preceded the death of their child and all that followed it, of all that was said and what was not said. For many parents explanations and interpretations ultimately lead back to them and foster a sense of self-blame for their child's death.

Initial reactions to a child's death will vary—from hysteria or rage to collapse or withdrawal. An environment that fosters and accepts all responses is helpful. Encouraging family members to come together at this time promotes communication among members. Questions, fears, and fantasies surface and are dealt with, increasing understanding of each other's responses. This is a time to assist the family in accepting the reality of the death. It becomes a time to see and confirm that their child is dead. No mistakes were made. If desired, it is also a time to begin the painful process of separation by saying good-bye. Parents may choose to hold their child, dress their child, talk to him or look at him, and become aware of the presence of death. Families will require space and time and permission to grieve openly and with support.

Usually families are confronted with a multitude of decisions at a time when decision making is most arduous. An autopsy may be requested or required, regardless of need or desire; parents' concerns and fears about the procedure will emerge. The child continues to be part of them and they continue to provide care to their child; the decision to submit their child to an autopsy is a painful one. Funeral and burial plans will also be made. Even though planning may be difficult for the parents, they should be encouraged to make these decisions. Often plans are made by well-meaning relatives or friends to save the parents from this difficult task; later, parents wish that they had exhibited more control and planned a service that met their needs to care about their child and assist them in their grief.

The caregiver serves as a resource person knowledgeable about community advocates and agencies that may be helpful to families in raising monies for the service, if needed. The caregiver may be helpful in locating a funeral director or local association of funeral directors who will assist the family with special needs. The family's choice can then be supported. It also helps to be familiar with the local death investigation process. In situations of sudden and unexpected death the medical examiner or coroner's office will typically be involved. Families can be informed of protocol and provided with concrete information and direction so that procedures will be anticipated. Knowledge about death certificates and public burial funds may be an immeasurable benefit to the family. Such information can be written down for families, who can refer to it for useful direction. Finally, local resources for information and counseling can be provided; particularly helpful will be the name of a parent contact from a helping organization that may also sponsor bereaved parent group meetings or telephone contact.

In working with the family members immediately following a child's death it is essential to support expressions of grief. The body provides a state of numbness. Expressions of grief need to be released from within the bereaved person. The form that these expressions take is varied. Caregivers will deal with their own personal fears and responses to another's pain and hopefully be able to allow any expression as acceptable as well as offer anticipatory guidance about subsequent grief behaviors. It also helps the family members to realize from the start that each individual grieves differently and may not feel the same at the same time.

Although the bereaved parent may feel that life is senseless and meaningless and that his own life means little, these expressions of powerlessness and guilt need to be differentiated from suicidal thoughts. It is different to feel that it would not matter if one fell out a window or stepped in front of a car than to plan one's own death. Although it is difficult to predict behavior, some clues of the parent at risk are outright sharing of the suicide plan, being alone without support, and putting one's life in order as though separating one's connections. It is imperative that a bereaved parent not leave the emergency room alone, leaving the dead child behind and leaving without human contact and support. In addition, some defined contract can be made with the family members for follow-up and a telephone number provided for the parents to call should they want to reach out for information or support.

If the child died suddenly or at home, it is critical for the caregiver to speak with the person who found the dead child. Agonal signs, or signs that relate to death itself, may be misinterpreted as neglectful behavior on this person's part because he has no recourse but to blame himself.

Also in this immediate period after the death of a child, it is helpful to assess the family's ability to sustain itself through the ensuing chaos. Usually someone will emerge as the natural leader and provide direction. Concrete and helpful information can be provided to this person. Lastly, one determines if support networks in the local community can be mobilized to assist the bereaved family.

Working with the family over time allows the caregiver to:

- explore issues,
- open communication, and
- offer information and provide anticipatory guidance.

The caregiver may explore with the family issues such as the meaning of their child to them; the disruption of their lives; their understanding of the cause and circumstances of the child's death; their impression of what they were told about their child's death; what they really think happened, since discrepancies between what they were told and what they think happened may exist; reactions from others—neighbors, police, ambulance and emergency room personnel, etc.—their immediate problems; and how they feel the caregiver can be helpful to them. The caregiver will support the family in exploration of critical issues for them by focusing on their strengths, fostering their abilities and decision-making capabilities. It is also important to gather together family members and other supportive people whom they identify as issues are raised and discussed.

To assist in opening communication within the family system, the caregiver looks for blocks in communication within the family. Are family members blaming each other or protecting each other from their own feelings or from difficult tasks? One member may be made a scapegoat or used as the focus for expressions of anger. The caregiver is mindful of the shattered sense of self and self-esteem that the parents may be experiencing. If there are surviving children in the family, the parents can be encouraged to take responsibility for these children and thereby foster the restoration of self-esteem. Specific concerns of siblings, which parents find most painful to deal with, are usually unresolved areas of pain for themselves. The caregiver asks questions that are helpful to the family in opening communication.

Anticipatory information about the wide range of normal grief reactions is helpful since there are few guideposts to assist bereaved parents in comprehending the nature of their grief. Issues related to blame, self-blame, blaming spouse, God, doctors, etc., are sought so that blame becomes recognizable, understood, and focused. In order to bear grief, parents need in some way to ask why their child died. Information is helpful in sorting out facts from distortions.

The family will need guidance in planning for what to expect tomorrow, the day after that, and next year. For instance, future episodes of acute grief are part of the normal grieving process, especially at significant times like the child's birthday, the anniversary of his death, other days or places that were special to the family, and the birth of subsequent children. The family will also need assistance in helping them cope with extended family members and community reactions. Sometimes feelings can be normalized if they can be anticipated—like the pain and jealous rage experienced at the sight of another's healthy baby, alive and well and living with his parents. Powerful grief responses follow a child's death whether sudden and unexpected or known and anticipated. The finality of death is always a shock. Emptiness cannot be erased by anticipation.

Information is helpful primarily as a way of preventing misinformation. Sometimes family members will gather more and more information as a way to defend themselves by intellectualizing their responses and distancing themselves from their feelings. Too much assistance runs the risk of becoming less than helpful and even rendering the parents helpless and unable to gather the energy to mobilize their own strengths and discover their own course of action. Working with the bereaved family is best accomplished through clarification of feelings and thoughts; promotion of congruent messages, feelings, and reactions that are in synchrony; and validation of the significance of all expressions of grief. The family is viewed as a vital system, not incapacitated and helpless, but capable and strong. In some way the family needs to know that tomorrow will be different from today. Grief has valleys, plateaus, and peaks. One does not get steadily better, but one moves through a process, experiencing the depths and heights of emotion. Pain does lessen with time, although it can return in an instant. Sharing memories helps to soothe and heal. Memories live.

The caregiver determines with the family when phases of the work together are completed. Grief needs time to be expressed and dealt with; it cannot be forced, particularly if someone needs to delay his grief. So many factors come together to influence specific grief responses; one's past experience with death, previous losses, how they are dealt with, one's sense of inner peace and control, and more. The need for solitude may be so strong or the anger of powerlessness so pervasive that the caregiver may be rejected or become the recipient of these reactions. The bereaved parents may be agitated because others expect them to return to normal living long before they are ready to pick up the pieces and restore some semblance of order in their lives. Death also precipitates other family problems, which demand attention before the family is free to grieve their lost member; dilemmas of poverty, medical problems, problems with housing are only a few influences that confound the process of grief.

Sometimes the bereaved need permission from others to enjoy themselves in spite of their sorrow. It is perfectly normal to want to feel happiness and be released from anguish—and still love and miss the dead child. The family lives with their dead child as he is always part of the family's identity, but they also live beyond him as time brings change and newness.

The caregiver offers to the family continuing availability, reflecting the long-lasting nature of family bereavement. It is essential for the caregiver to remain available to the family. It may take months or years before a family can raise and deal with issues related to the child's death. For others, reaching out requires energy that is now dissipated. Outreach to the bereaved family is essential.

In working with bereaved families the caregiver comes to realize that more is shared than is different. We all are survivors ultimately. The caregiver opens himself to the impact of death in his own life, demystifies death, and becomes committed to providing care to survivors.

Reference

Donnelly, K.F. *Recovering from the loss of a child.* New York: Macmillan, 1982. (Part I presents first-hand accounts of how people have managed to survive an excruciating bereavement—the death of a child. Part II describes organizations that help bereaved families and lists them in directory form.)

Suggested Reading

Cassel, E.J. The nature of suffering and the goals of medicine. *New England Journal of Medicine,* March 18, 1982, 306, 639-645.

On the Death of His Child[*]

O brightness of my bright eyes, how art thou? Without thee my days are
dark; without me how art thou?

My house is a house of mourning in thine absence; thou hast made
thine abode beneath the dust: how art thou?

The couch and pillow of thy sleep is on thorns and brambles: O thou
whose cheeks and body were as jasmine, how art thou?

Faydí (d. 1595)
Translated from Persian
by E.G. Browne

[*]Reprinted with permission from Cambridge University Press. From A Literary History of
Persia.

Appendix

Books about Death
for Children
and Parents

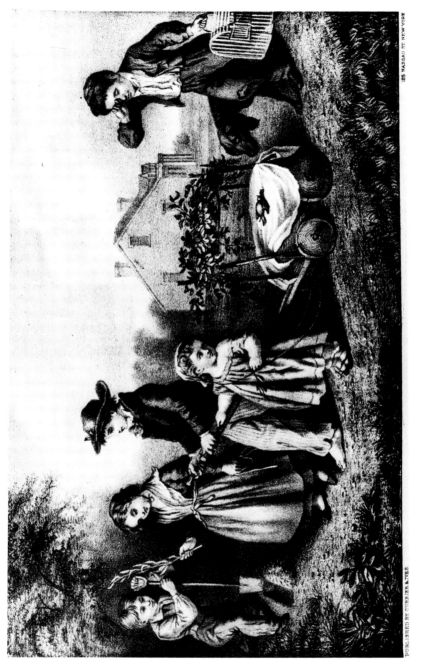

CURRIER AND IVES, © 1872-1874. *The Burial of the Bird.* Lithograph. 8 × 10, B&W (Reprinted with permission from the collections of Henry Ford Museum, The Edison Institute, Dearborn, Michigan, neg. no. B3636.)

The following listing of children's books about death is by no means exhaustive. It contains a few that introduce young children to the experience of death and to the myriad of feelings that children have in response to this important event in their lives. These references for the preschool and young school-age child present the theme of death gently and poignantly through the death of a beloved pet.

The remaining references for older children consider specifically a close friend or sibling's death and the family's response to this loss.

Included for the parent is a brief listing of specially selected books and pamphlets that offer guidelines for talking with children about death and their feeling responses.

Books for Young Children and Parents Dealing with Death through Loss of an Animal

The Dead Bird by Margaret Wise Brown. Addison-Wesley, Reading, Massachusetts, 1958.
(*3-5 years*) This simply told story is about a group of children who discover a bird, realize it is dead, and prepare to bury it.

The Tenth Good Thing about Barney by Judith Viorst. Antheneum Publishers, New York, 1971.
(*5-8 years*) This is a poignant narrative by a small boy of his feelings of sadness when his pet cat dies. The boy and his parents bury the pet and discuss the warm memories that they have of Barney.

Accident by Carol Carrick. Seabury Press, New York, 1976.
(*6-8 years*) Christopher is helped by his father to express his grief when his dog Badger is killed by a truck. Together they search for a special rock to mark his grave.

Books for Older Children and Young Adolescents
on Death of a Sibling or Close Friend

A Taste of Blackberries by Doris B. Smith. Thomas Y. Crowell
  Company, 1973.
(*8-9 years*) The author conveys the experience and feelings of an
eight-year-old boy whose best friend Jamie dies accidentally. The boy
and his family, along with Jamie's family, deal with the myriad of
questions and feelings engendered by this unexpected event.

Confessions of an Only Child by Norma Klein. Pantheon
  Books, New York, 1974.
(*8-12 years*) When Antonia, who is nine-years-old, anticipates having a new sibling with which to share her parents and home, she has
mixed feelings. However, when that baby dies, she is very sad.

The Magic Moth by Virginia Lee. Seabury Press, New York,
  1972.
(*10-12 years*) This is the poignant story of a family of seven whose
middle child, 10-year-old Maryanne, dies at home from an irrepara-
ble cardiac defect. The parents handle the death and the responses of
the surviving children sensitively.

Little Women by Louise May Alcott. Macmillan, New York,
  1962 (originally 1869).
(*10-14 years*) This favorite classic presents the story of Beth's invalid-
ism and eventual death. Interwoven throughout are Beth's own sense
of her dying and the responses of her family and friends.

Beat the Turtle Drum by Constance C. Greene. The Viking
  Press, New York, 1976.
(*10-14 years*) In this touching story, the effect of the sudden death of
the 11-year-old child on her older sister and parents is told with
warmth and sensitivity.

Bridge to Terabithia by Katherine Paterson. Thomas Y. Crowell Company, 1977.
(*10-14 years*) This portrays the grief of Jess, a 10-year-old boy in rural Virginia, who becomes close friends with a newcomer, Leslie. Leslie dies while trying to reach their hideaway, Terabithia, during a storm.

Guidelines for Parents

Explaining Death to Children by Earl A. Grollman. Beacon Press, Boston, 1967.
This is a simple and straightforward presentation of children's concerns and questions about death and adult answers and responses.

Talking about Death: A Dialogue between Parent and Child by Earl A. Grollman. Beacon Press, Boston, 1976.
To be read before and then with one's child, this book contains a story about the death of a grandfather, which can be adapted easily. The story is followed by a text directed at helping parents understand children's concepts of death at different ages.

Talking to Children about Death by National Institute of Mental Health, DHEW Publication No. 79-838 (a free publication).
This is a guide to understanding children's reactions to death, with some ways to support and help the child with the experience of loss.

About Dying by Sara Bonnett Stein. Walker and Company, New York, 1974.
This is a book to be read by children and families together. Death is introduced straightforwardly and gently in doses tolerable to children of different ages.

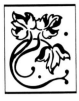

Index

Italic page numbers indicate illustrations.

About the Authors

Joan Hagan Arnold, R.N., M.A.

Assistant Professor, School of Nursing, Adelphi University; Consultant, New York City Information and Counseling Program for Sudden Infant Death and doctoral candidate Department of Research and Theory Development in Nursing Science, New York University.

Penelope Buschman Gemma, R.N., M.S., C.S.

Administrative Nurse Clinician, Babies Hospital, Columbia-Presbyterian Medical Center; Associate in Clinical Nursing, School of Nursing, Columbia University, New York.